Ear, Nose and Throat

THIRD EDITION

and Head and Neck Surgery

AN ILLUSTRATED COLOUR TEXT

Commissioning Editor: Michael Parkinson
Project Development Manager: Joan Morrison
Project Manager: Nancy Arnott
Designer: Erik Bigland
Illustration Manager: Bruce Hogarth
Illustration Design: Cactus Design

THIRD EDITION

Ear, nose and throat

and head and neck surgery

AN ILLUSTRATED COLOUR TEXT

R.S. DHILLON FRCS
Hon. Professor, Middlesex University, London
Consultant ENT, Head and Neck Surgeon
Northwick Park Hospital and Clinical Research Centre
Middlesex, London, UK

C.A. EAST FRCS
Consultant ENT, Head and Neck Surgeon
The Royal National Throat, Nose and Ear Hospital
Institute of Laryngology and Otology
The Royal Free Hampstead NHS Trust, London, UK

with contributions by

A. NARULA FRCS
Hon. Professor, Middlesex University, London
Consultant ENT Surgeon
St Mary's NHS Trust, London, UK

G. SANDHU FRCS
Consultant ENT Surgeon
The Hammersmith Hospitals NHS Trust and
The Royal National Throat, Nose and Ear Hospital, London, UK

J-P. JEANNON FRCS
Consultant ENT Surgeon
Guy's and St Thomas' NHS Foundation Trust, London, UK

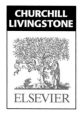

CHURCHILL
LIVINGSTONE

ELSEVIER

EDINBURGH   LONDON   NEW YORK   OXFORD   PHILADELPHIA   ST LOUIS   SYDNEY   TORONTO   2006

CHURCHILL
LIVINGSTONE
ELSEVIER

© Longman Group UK Limited 1994
© Churchill Livingstone, a division of Harcourt Brace and Company Limited 1999
© Harcourt Publishers Limited 2001
© 2006 Elsevier Limited. All rights reserved.

First edition 1994
Second edition 1999
Third edition 2006

ISBN-13: 978-0-443-07311-3
ISBN-10: 0-443-07311-2

British Library Cataloguing in Publication Data
A catalogue record for this book is available from the British Library.

Library of Congress Cataloging in Publication Data
A catalog record for this book is available from the Library of Congress.

ELSEVIER your source for books, journals and multimedia in the health sciences
www.elsevierhealth.com

Working together to grow libraries in developing countries
www.elsevier.com | www.bookaid.org | www.sabre.org
ELSEVIER BOOK AID International Sabre Foundation

The publisher's policy is to use **paper manufactured from sustainable forests**

Printed in China

Foreword

It is a testament to the foresight of the authors and publishers that *Ear, Nose and Throat and Head and Neck Surgery* continues to be such a success, not only nationally in the UK but also worldwide. The text has found a place in many medical schools and has acted as a primer for general practitioners, trainees in ENT and nurse practitioners. In the era of electronic publications, the 'topic on a double page' format has proved that many still enjoy reading from a traditional textbook.

The third edition has changed in recognition of the fact that, with increasing subspecialization in head and neck surgery, there is a need for subspecialist input. The book thus covers the basic broad spectrum of head and neck surgery with more detailed input from experts in their field on individual topics.

The concept of the third edition is still to provide concise, easy to assimilate information for all those who deal with diseases in the head and neck: ENT, facial plastic, maxillofacial and general practitioners. I believe this text will continue to inform and hopefully inspire many more in this interesting and expanding area of medicine.

London
2006

Tony Wright
Professor of Otorhinolaryngology
Institute of Laryngology and Otology
University College
London

Preface

The third edition of *Ear, Nose and Throat and Head and Neck Surgery* is still primarily intended for medical students, general practitioners, including those with a special interest in head and neck diseases, and nursing and paramedical staff. Feedback over the years has also highlighted that the book is valuable to other clinicians treating diseases of the head and neck; in particular, it has acted as a primer for junior ENT specialists both nationally and internationally.

We both recognize that, with increasing diversification and subspecialization, help was needed in achieving an up-to-date textbook that covers the vast range of diseases related to ENT and head and neck surgery. The basic style of the book has remained the same, wih topics dealt with in double-page spreads and the content presented in a mixture of text, line drawings, tables, colour illustrations and key point summaries. This 'educational unit' approach enhances accessibility and is extremely useful in revision. ENT and head and neck surgery has now become a major speciality within the surgical domain. It encompasses not only the time-honoured ear, nose and throat but also facial, aesthetic and reconstructive surgery, head and neck and skull base surgery. It has a non-surgical branch in audiology – audiological medicine – that bears the same relationship to ENT surgery as neurology to neurosurgery and cardiology to cardiac surgery.

We have endeavoured to cover the new developments and extensions within the speciality, including those of cochlear implantation for the deaf, investigations of snoring and sleep apnoea, and airway management. The more common disorders are covered in detail in both diagnostic and management areas; however, the operative details have been kept to a minimum as we recognize that these are particularly relevant to dedicated ENT and head and neck specialists.

London
2006

R. S. Dhillon
C.A. East

Acknowledgements

We are extremely grateful to numerous friends and colleagues who have assisted us in completing this book.

We must thank Mr Richards Williams who, at the inception of this text, was Director of the Ferens Institute of Otolaryngology at University College London Medical School and allowed us free rein of the excellent facilities available there. The Ferens is now part of the Institute of Laryngology and Otology, University College London.

We are delighted that Antony Narula, Guri Sandhu and Jean-Pierre Jeannon have written significant contributions to the third edition.

From the First Edition in 1994. Many colleagues have helped with advice and illustations. These include: Martin Bailey, Tony Wright, David Howard, Robin Kantor, David Katz, Peter Phelps, Jim Fairley, Charles Croft, Saleem Goolamali, Edward Townsend, Steve Watt-Smith, J.N. Blau, Glynn Lloyd, Ian Colquhoun and Arnold Maran. Additionally, thanks go to the Institute of Laryngology and Otology Medical Photography Department and David Fenton for Figure 3(a), page 106 (*Nail in Disease* published by Butterworth Heinemann) and Michael Dilkes for Figures 3(a) and (b), page 47. Particular thanks to Garry Glover, whose slide collection was invaluable.

Our appreciation is due to our secretaries for their patient typing. Thanks to the publishing team including Michael Parkinson and Joan Morrison, and finally to everyone who has encouraged this project and bought copies of our book!

London   R. S. Dhillon
2006   C. A. East

Contents

The Ear

Basic concepts

Anatomy and physiology

Structurally, the ear has three parts (Fig. 1):

- the external ear
- the middle ear
- the inner ear.

The external ear

The external ear includes the pinna, external auditory meatus and tympanic membrane. The outer part has a cartilage skeleton, and the deep part is bony. Both are covered by skin. The skin on the outer part contains hair follicles and wax glands, but these elements are absent in the deep meatus. Canal skin migrates outwards from the deep meatus, but does not desquamate until it reaches the junction with the cartilaginous meatus. This normal mechanism may be disturbed by injudicious use of cotton buds.

The eardrum is the window of the middle ear and is divided into the pars tensa and pars flaccida. The main landmark on the drum is the malleus handle (Fig. 2).

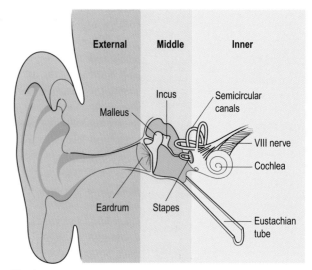

Fig. 1 **Anatomy of the ear.** For descriptive purposes the ear is divided into three parts: the external, the middle and the inner ear.

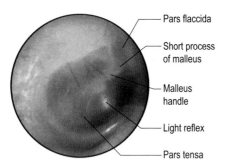

Fig. 2 **A normal right eardrum.**

The middle ear

The middle ear is an air-containing space connected to the nasopharynx via the Eustachian tube. It acts as an impedance matching device to transfer sound energy efficiently from air to a fluid medium in the cochlea (Fig. 3). The middle ear space, including the mastoid air cells, is closely related to the temporal lobe, cerebellum, jugular bulb and labyrinth of the inner ear. The space contains three ossicles (the malleus, incus and stapes) which transmit sound vibrations from the eardrum to the cochlea. The middle ear also contains two small muscles and is traversed by the facial nerve before it exits the skull.

The inner ear

The inner ear comprises a dense bony capsule containing a membranous labyrinth which forms the cochlea, vestibule and semicircular canals.

The membranous part is surrounded by fluid, called perilymph, and is sealed from the middle ear by the stapes footplate and round window membrane.

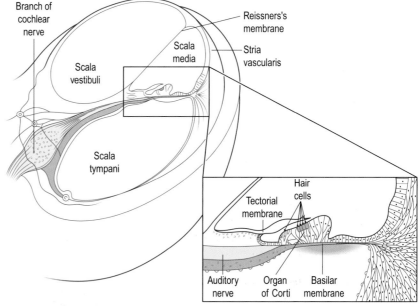

Fig. 3 **Section through the cochlea.** Hair cells in the organ of Corti transform mechanical energy (vibration) into electrical impulses.

The membranous part itself contains fluid called endolymph. The cochlea contains the organ of hearing which is connected by the auditory nerve to the brain stem (Fig. 3).

Normal hearing depends on transmission of sound via a vibrating tympanic membrane through a mobile ossicular chain to the cochlea. Displacement of the basilar membrane and movement of the hair cells cause an organized volley of electrical discharge in the eighth nerve, perceived as sound in the cerebral cortex.

The vestibule and semicircular canals form the peripheral balance organ. These have connections to the cerebellum and the eyes, and are important in the maintenance of posture and the ability to keep the eyes fixed when the head is moving.

Symptoms and signs

Symptoms

History taking in ear complaints should be brief but thorough. Table 1 provides a reference guide of the major points which should be covered. The otological symptoms are discussed in greater detail later in this section, but it is important to establish the predominant complaint and whether it affects one or both ears.

Table 1 **Major points in history taking in patients with an otological complaint**	
Otological	**Nasal**
Hearing loss — onset and rate of progression	Obstruction, discharge, etc.
Otalgia	**Drugs**
Otorrhoea	Ototoxic agents (e.g. aminoglycosides)
Tinnitus	
Imbalance	**Family history**
	Hearing loss
Noise exposure	
Previous ear surgery	

Signs

Satisfactory examination cannot be undertaken without adequate lighting. Battery auriscopes with a fibre or glass ring light give a coaxial beam with bright uniform illumination. A pneumatic attachment tests the mobility of the eardrum (Fig. 4).

The pinna should be examined for scars and signs of crusting or weeping. Before introducing the auriscope, the ear canal must be straightened by elevating the pinna upwards and backwards (Fig. 4). The condition of the ear canal should be noted before the eardrum is examined. If an adequate seal of the canal is achieved by the speculum, gentle pressure on the pneumatic bulb will move the eardrum if the middle ear contains air. This is helpful in distinguishing perforations from thin or translucent segments.

A complete examination also involves viewing the Eustachian tube orifice in the nasopharynx.

Clinical tests of hearing

A sympathetic approach is important to overcome embarrassment or denial with potential hearing problems. Whisper and voice tests are of little value unless performed in a quiet room with a sound pressure level meter placed near the patient. The following tests are more useful.

Tuning fork tests

Tuning fork tests distinguish between conductive and sensorineural hearing loss, but are of limited value in children. Two tests are usually employed using a 512 Hz fork. The fork is sounded by striking the tines against the patella or elbow.

Rinne test. The Rinne test compares air conduction (AC – hearing via ear canal and middle ear) with bone conduction (BC – direct transmission to the inner ear via the mastoid process). The examiner holds the fork by the ear canal and then places it on the mastoid process using gentle counterpressure with the other hand. The patient is asked which position of the fork sounds louder – in front of the ear or touching the mastoid (Fig. 5).

Sound is normally heard better by air conduction than bone conduction (Rinne-positive). Disease in the external or middle ear, producing a conductive deafness, will reverse the test result (Rinne-negative).

Weber test. The Weber test is more sensitive than the Rinne test. The tuning fork is placed on the forehead, in the midline and sound waves are transmitted to both ears equally via the skull. A conductive deafness in one ear causes the sound to be heard on the same side. A sensorineural deafness causes the sound to be heard on the opposite side.

The interpretation of the tuning fork tests in relation to the type of hearing loss is shown in Figure 5. Avoid the false Rinne-negative by adequately masking the contralateral ear.

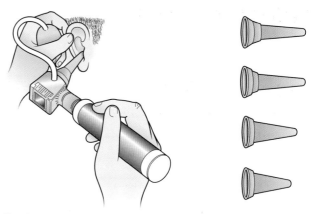

Fig. 4 **Inserting the auriscope.** The pinna is elevated upwards and backwards. The instrument should be gripped like a pencil.

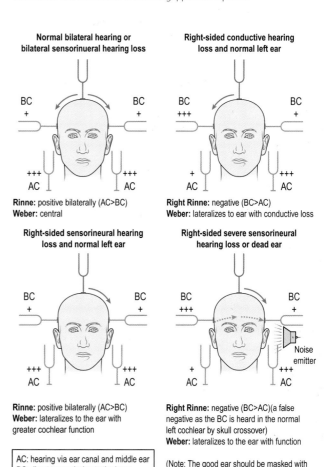

Normal bilateral hearing or bilateral sensorinueral hearing loss

Rinne: positive bilaterally (AC>BC)
Weber: central

Right-sided conductive hearing loss and normal left ear

Right Rinne: negative (BC>AC)
Weber: lateralizes to ear with conductive loss

Right-sided sensorineural hearing loss and normal left ear

Rinne: positive bilaterally (AC>BC)
Weber: lateralizes to the ear with greater cochlear function

Right-sided severe sensorineural hearing loss or dead ear

Noise emitter

Right Rinne: negative (BC>AC)(a false negative as the BC is heard in the normal left cochlear by skull crossover)
Weber: lateralizes to ear with function

AC: hearing via ear canal and middle ear
BC: direct transmission to the inner ear via mastoid process
+ subjective loudness

Weber test   Rinne test

(Note: The good ear should be masked with a noise emitter and the test repeated. The right-sided BC will be greatly reduced or absent.)

Fig. 5 **The interpretation of tuning fork tests.** These tests are invalidated if the ear canals are not free of wax debris.

Basic concepts

- Establish the precise otological complaint from the patient.
- Nasopharyngeal pathology can cause secondary ear disease so always examine this region.
- Beware the false Rinne-negative in cases of severe unilateral sensorineural hearing loss.
- A dead ear must be recognized before any surgery.

Audiometry, vestibulometry and radiology

Until the advent of audiometers, hearing was tested exclusively by the examiner's voice and tuning forks. Modern hearing tests are performed in soundproofed rooms using high precision electronic audiological equipment. All tests require cooperation from the patient. Those tests requiring patient response are termed *subjective tests*, while those not requiring patient response are termed *objective*.

Audiometry

Subjective tests

Pure tone audiograms are a standard means of recording hearing levels. Using headphones, each ear is tested individually for air conduction and, if necessary, bone conduction thresholds. The results are usually plotted as a graph. A result of 0 dB (decibels) is the average normal threshold for hearing in young adults (Fig. 1).

Speech audiometry is a more sophisticated test. Phonetically balanced words are presented at different sound intensities and the number of correct answers is expressed as a percentage score. This is a useful test for evaluating hearing aids.

Objective tests

Impedance audiometry is an extremely useful test in the diagnosis of middle ear disease and some types of sensorineural hearing loss. By varying the pressure in the external ear canal, the compliance (i.e. mobility) of the eardrum may be calculated by the degree of sound reflected from a probe tone. This is very useful when screening for middle ear effusions, particularly in children, and for assessing Eustachian tube function (p. 7). It can also test the integrity of the middle ear mechanism and the auditory reflex arc (stapedius reflex).

Electric response audiometry (ERA) (Fig. 2) is another objective test. An evoked potential in the eighth nerve, brain stem or auditory cortex may be recorded using skin electrodes following acoustic stimulation of the cochlea. This principle is used to objectively assess hearing thresholds where the standard tests are not applicable, e.g. babies, handicapped people and suspected malingerers.

Oto-acoustic emissions testing is a useful screening test for neonatal sensorineural loss where the middle ear function is normal.

Hearing assessment in young children

From birth to about 6 months, the 'gold standard' method of testing is by electric response audiometry (see above). From 6 months to about 18 months, a child will turn to a noise, e.g. a rattle. This *distraction test* is performed by two observers and is a basic screening test performed on all children. From 2 years, various *conditioning or cooperation tests* are employed using free field noises, e.g. placing a peg in a basket after hearing the noise. It is not until the age of 3–4 years that headphones can be used to independently test each ear.

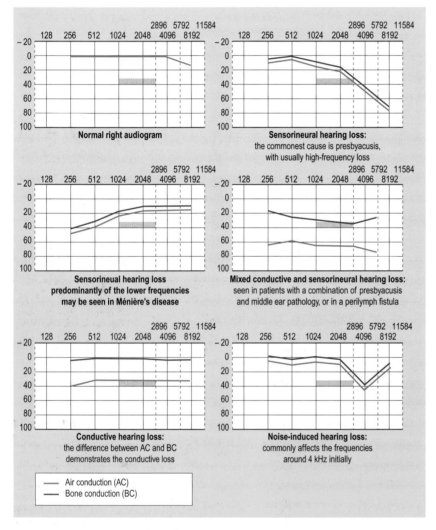

Fig. 1 **A series of typical pure tone audiograms of the right ear.** Hearing level (dBISO) is plotted on the vertical axis; frequency (Hz) is plotted on the horizontal axis. Air conduction (AC) signals are fed through headphones. Bone conduction (BC) signals are transmitted via a vibrator placed on the mastoid process.

The graphs are labelled:
- Normal right audiogram
- Sensorineural hearing loss: the commonest cause is presbyacusis, with usually high-frequency loss
- Sensorineual hearing loss predominantly of the lower frequencies may be seen in Ménière's disease
- Mixed conductive and sensorineural hearing loss: seen in patients with a combination of presbyacusis and middle ear pathology, or in a perilymph fistula
- Conductive hearing loss: the difference between AC and BC demonstrates the conductive loss
- Noise-induced hearing loss: commonly affects the frequencies around 4 kHz initially

Legend:
— Air conduction (AC)
— Bone conduction (BC)

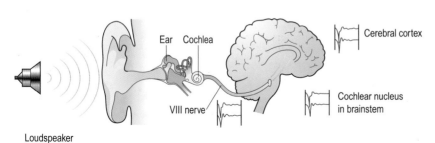

Fig. 2 **Evoked response audiometry.** The response evoked by a sound stimulus can be recorded at a specific site along the auditory pathway, e.g. eighth nerve, brainstem or the cortex.

Labels: Ear, Cochlea, Cerebral cortex, VIII nerve, Cochlear nucleus in brainstem, Loudspeaker

Vestibulometry

The vestibule has three parts: the utricle, the saccule and the semicircular canals (Fig. 1, p. 2). Each vestibule tonically discharges information to the brain regarding head position, and linear and angular acceleration. This information is part of the general proprioceptive input (joint, tendon, skin and ocular inputs). Dysequilibrium may be the result of an abnormal input from any part of the proprioceptive sensors, or a dysfunction of the central nervous connection secondary to disease, e.g. ischaemia or demyelination.

Stimulation or destruction of one labyrinth produces nystagmus, an hallucination of movement (vertigo) and a feeling of nausea. Nystagmus associated with peripheral vestibular disease produces a horizontal rhythmic eye movement with a slow and fast component. The direction of nystagmus is named according to the fast component. Nystagmus in directions other than horizontal is associated with central vestibular disorders.

Tests
The functional status of the peripheral vestibular system can be tested in a variety of ways. These include:

- positional test
- fistula test
- caloric test
- rotation tests and electronystagmography.

Positional test
From an erect sitting position on a couch, the patient lies flat with the head turned to one side and below horizontal (Fig. 3). The onset of any vertigo is noted and the eyes are observed for nystagmus. The feeling of movement and the nystagmus, if present, are allowed to settle before the patient sits upright. The manoeuvre is repeated with the head to the opposite side. This test may help distinguish vertigo caused by peripheral (otological) as opposed to central pathologies.

Fistula test
If there is otoscopic evidence of middle ear disease in a patient with vertigo, this simple test may be applied.

A calorific effect is induced by either compressing the tragus, or by using an otoscope with a pneumatic bulb. A feeling of imbalance or vertigo, sometimes accompanied by nystagmus, indicates an abnormal communication between the middle ear and vestibular labyrinth (a positive sign).

Caloric test
Cold (30°C) or warm (44°C) water irrigation of the ear canal stimulates the labyrinth and will induce nystagmus in normal ears. Cold water produces nystagmus to the opposite side to that tested and warm the reverse. (Remember COWS – Cold Opposite, Warm Same – for direction of nystagmus). This test indicates the presence or absence of function in a particular labyrinth.

Rotation tests and electronystagmography
Rotational tests assess the vestibular response to angular acceleration by measuring nystagmus from surface electrodes around the ocular muscles. Various other tests of eye pivot, optical fixation and suppression of nystagmus may be recorded by electronystagmography. These investigations give information about central mechanisms and disorders of the vestibular nuclei in the brainstem (p. 20).

Posturography
Modern balance-testing equipment allows the separation of visual and/or proprioceptive input to balance. This further helps to delineate the causes of vertigo but is not yet widely available.

Radiology

Imaging of the temporal bone is now done with CT or magnetic resonance imaging (MRI). Plain radiographs only provide evidence of gross disease and their interpretation may be difficult. Clouding of mastoid air cells may be seen in acute mastoiditis. Disease which produces significant bony erosion may be shown on plain X-rays, e.g. carcinoma of the middle ear.

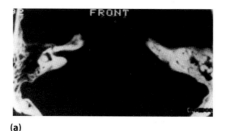
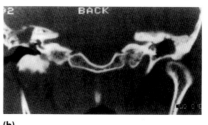
(a) (b)

Fig. 4 **Axial (a) and coronal (b) CT of the temporal bone.** The patient has vertigo from a middle ear cholesteatoma eroding the left lateral semicircular canal. The mastoid air cell system is opaque.

Modern CT scanning and MRI are now widely used to provide information on otitis media with complications, and in the diagnosis of acoustic neuromas (Figs 4 & 5). MRI is particularly useful in assessing the extent of vascular lesions such as glomus jugulare tumours, and in visualizing the acoustic nerve.

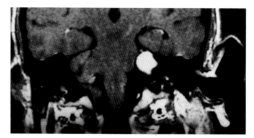

Fig. 5 **Large acoustic neuroma with early compression of the brainstem.** The lesion is enhanced by injection of gadolinium contrast into a peripheral vein.

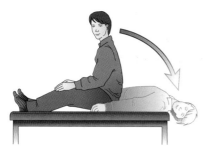

Fig. 3 **'Positional testing' in cases of vertigo.**

Audiometry, vestibulometry and radiology

- Correctly performed pure tone audiograms are the most reliable method of assessing hearing thresholds.
- Electric response audiometry may be required in assessing the thresholds in very young infants and others who are unable to respond to subjective audiometric tests.
- Impedance audiometry is extremely useful in assessing the presence of middle ear effusions.
- A patient with a positive fistula test in the presence of chronic ear disease requires urgent otological referral.

Hearing loss — General introduction and childhood aetiology

General introduction

A hearing loss, as mentioned previously, can be either conductive, sensorineural or mixed. Any disease affecting the outer or middle ear will produce a conductive deafness. Sensorineural loss results from damage to the cochlea or eighth nerve. The degree of hearing loss can be quantified on an audiogram with the thresholds of hearing quoted in decibels (p. 4).

Table 1 lists the commonest causes of hearing loss. Most of those leading to a conductive deafness will be evident from history, otoscopy, tuning fork tests and audiometry. However, the aetiology of sensorineural loss is frequently unclear. In these cases, specific points in the history should be determined. These points are listed in Table 2.

In general terms, a conductive hearing loss is amenable to surgery. However, a common feature of sensorineural deafness is loss of hair cells from the organ of Corti. Hair cells are not replaced, thus sensory deafness is usually permanent. Sensorineural losses often display predominantly high tone loss on audiometry as the hair cells responding to high frequencies are most susceptible to damage.

Hearing loss in children

Deafness is an impairment to communication at any age, but children born with a hearing loss have a major handicap in developing communication. Therefore, early detection and management are required for adequate speech and language development.

The incidence of severe sensorineural deafness is about 1 in 1000. Half of these children have an hereditary type of deafness (Fig. 1). The others have hearing losses resulting from acquired causes. Even mild degrees of hearing loss, either conductive or sensorineural, can impair learning ability.

Childhood hearing loss should be suspected in certain groups of individuals (Table 3). Children falling

Table 1 Aetiology of hearing loss

Cause	Conductive hearing loss	Sensorineural hearing loss
Congenital	Atresia of ear, ossicular abnormalities	Prenatal: genetic, rubella
Acquired	External: wax, otitis externa, foreign body	Perinatal: hypoxia, jaundice
	Middle ear: middle ear effusion, chronic otitis (cholesteatoma, perforated drum), otosclerosis, traumatic perforation of drum (ossicular disruption)	Trauma: noise, head injury, surgery
		Inflammatory: chronic otitis, meningitis, measles, mumps, syphilis
		Degenerative: presbyacusis
		Ototoxicity: aminoglycosides, cytotoxics
		Neoplastic: acoustic neuroma
		Idiopathic: Ménière's disease, sudden deafness

Table 2 Points to cover in clinical history of a patient presenting with hearing loss

Onset and rate of progression of hearing loss
Pain or discharge
Tinnitus
Imbalance
Excessive noise exposure
Drug history — ototoxic agents
Family history

Table 4 History taking in childhood hearing loss

General development and milestones
Age first word uttered
Extent of vocabulary
Verbal comprehension — Does he or she understand you?
Attention span and concentration
Social background and interactions
Family history of hearing loss

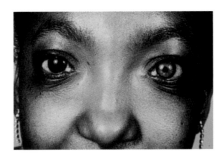

Fig. 1 **Waardenburg's syndrome.** This is a hereditary syndrome with sensorineural hearing loss. Other features include heterochromia iridian (different coloured irises), wide nasal bridge and a white forelock (not illustrated).

Table 3 The childhood groups at risk of suffering from hearing loss

Birth factors
— prematurity
— very low birth weight
— intraventricular haemorrhage
— neonatal jaundice
— aminoglycoside administration
Failed distraction test
Parental suspicion of hearing loss
Abnormal speech and language development
Parents or siblings with hearing loss

into these risk categories should be referred to an audiological physician or otologist for audiometric assessment. This is often a multidisciplinary approach using teachers of the deaf and speech therapists in the same clinic. If a hearing loss can be overcome at an early age, particularly severe sensorineural losses, there is a greater chance the child can attend an ordinary school. Where an hereditary loss is confirmed, a geneticist may advise on risks to future children.

History taking from the parents should concentrate on establishing the answers to specific questions, as well as making a general otological assessment (Table 4). Most hearing problems relate to middle ear disease. However, sensorineural deafness may coexist.

Children with a profound hearing loss should be fitted with an aid at the earliest possible opportunity after diagnosis. Great perseverance is needed with aiding, particularly in the first 2 years of life. Close observation by otologists, audiological physicians and teachers, with repeated assessments of hearing levels while aided, will give the best chance of normal development of speech and language.

Otitis media with effusion (OME; glue ear)

OME is the commonest cause of acquired conductive hearing loss in children. The true incidence is unknown, but up to 60% of children in their first year may have middle ear effusions which are clinically asymptomatic. The peak clinical age

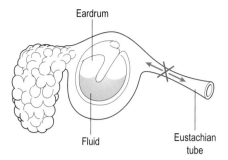

Fig. 2 **Eustachian tube dysfunction resulting in defective middle ear ventilation.** This can be due to a variety of causes and results in a middle ear effusion.

group is 2–6 years, where about 30% of children suffer effusions. By the age of 11 the incidence has dropped to about 2%. There is a seasonal variation in the disease, associated with upper respiratory tract infections which are more common in October to March in the northern hemisphere.

The effusion in the middle ear may be serous, mucoid or thick (glue). The aetiology is usually *Eustachian tube dysfunction*, where normal ventilation of the middle ear is disturbed (Fig. 2). **A diagnosis of chronic otitis media with effusion is made when fluid is present behind the eardrum for 12 weeks or more.**

Clinical features

Children with OME usually present with hearing loss or recurrent otalgia. Children with a cleft palate or Down syndrome have a higher incidence of middle ear effusions. The otoscopic features of OME are characteristic (Fig. 3).

The hearing loss is conductive and may fluctuate down to as much as 40 dB. Tympanometry produces a flat trace, indicating an immobile drum (Fig. 4).

Treatment

There is as yet no effective long-term medical treatment for established OME. Short-term improvements with antibiotics are not sustained. Decongestant mixtures are ineffective. If the effusion persists, surgery may be required to restore hearing. Removal of the adenoids reduces the incidence of recurrent effusions. Myringotomy, aspiration of fluid and insertion of a ventilation tube (grommet) immediately restores the hearing (Fig. 5). Grommets may remain in the drum for up to 12 months before being extruded. After grommet extrusion some children require

reinsertion due to recurrent or persisting middle ear effusions.

Following grommet extrusion, it is common to see tympanosclerosis (white patches) in the eardrum. This type of white patch does not impair hearing.

Chronic failure of the Eustachian tube to function normally results in persisting middle ear effusion and thinning of the tympanic membrane. The eardrum may collapse onto the ossicles, producing a retraction pocket. Long-term ventilation may be necessary to prevent progressive retraction from the low middle ear pressure and subsequent development of chronic suppurative otitis media with cholesteatoma.

Otorrhoea after grommets

Grommets may become infected, producing a mucoid discharge. This should be mopped away and anti-inflammatory drops instilled. Massaging the tragus will allow the drops to penetrate the grommet lumen. Antibiotic eardrops are not recommended except under specialist supervision. Oral antibiotics may also be necessary if the discharge follows an upper respiratory tract infection. Persistent otorrhoea will necessitate removal of the grommet.

Children with grommets should not be prevented from participating in swimming activities. Infection is uncommon and usually readily treated.

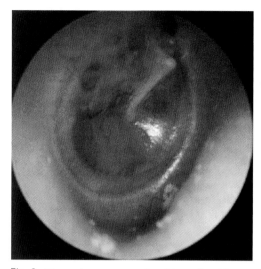

Fig. 3 **Otoscopic appearance in otitis media with effusion (OME).** The handle and short process of the malleus are brought into relief due to retraction of the eardrum. There is a slightly yellow appearance to the eardrum due to the middle ear effusion.

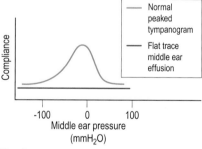

Fig. 4 **Impedance tympanometry.** This is an excellent method for detecting the presence of middle ear effusions. A flat compliance is seen in cases of otitis media with effusion.

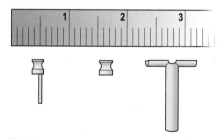

Fig. 5 **Types of grommets (middle ear ventilation tubes).** The variety of designs are numerous in an attempt to prevent too rapid an extrusion from the eardrum and to assist in insertion.

Hearing loss in children

- Childhood hearing loss needs early detection to maximize speech and language acquisition.
- Screening at 7–8 months is mandatory. Test failure requires early referral.
- Neonatal screening with oto-acoustic emissions is recommended.
- Middle ear effusions are common, and may be detected by pneumatic otoscopy.
- OME may present with otalgia, or may be asymptomatic until hearing loss is suspected.
- Insertion of grommets is required for persistent otitis media with effusion.
- Otorrhoea due to infected grommets usually resolves with topical treatments.

Hearing loss — Adult aetiology

The commonest causes of hearing loss in adults are wax impaction and presbyacusis. However, there are a number of other diseases in which hearing loss is the primary complaint, although often with other associated otological symptoms.

Conductive hearing loss

The aetiology of adult conductive hearing loss may be due to pathology of the ear canal, the eardrum or the middle ear.

Ear canal

Wax production varies between individuals and races. Blind attempts to remove wax with cotton buds usually results in impaction. Wax may be properly removed by syringing the ear or with a blunt hook (p. 25). Preliminary softening can be achieved with sodium bicarbonate eardrops three times a day, or hydrogen peroxide. Rarely, excessive accumulations of desquamated skin and wax in the deepest part of the external meatus can expand and erode the ear canal. This is termed *keratosis obturans*, and an anaesthetic may be required to remove it.

The external canal may be narrowed by bony exostoses predisposing to keratin accumulation (Fig. 1). These exostoses often occur in swimmers and require no treatment unless they cause external otitis or hearing deficits.

Eardrum and middle ear

Perforations of the eardrum can occur from trauma and acute or chronic otitis media (Fig. 2). The degree of hearing loss depends on the site of the perforation and the extent of middle ear disease.

Perforations from simple chronic otitis media where the mastoid is not diseased may be repaired by a tympanoplasty procedure using a graft (temporalis fascia). Ossicular discontinuity may also be treated surgically. Traumatic perforations, e.g. blow to the ear, invariably heal spontaneously if the ear is kept dry.

Adults may suffer with middle ear effusions, although less commonly than in children. Investigations should rule out sinusitis, or nasopharyngeal tumours blocking the Eustachian tube (Fig. 2, p. 7).

Otosclerosis is a disease where new bone growth occurs in the capsule of the inner ear. This may fix the footplate of the stapes. Hearing loss characteristically develops in the *young* adult and is usually conductive (p. 3), although the otoscopic appearance of the eardrum is normal. Pregnancy can accelerate the symptoms, suggesting an hormonal association with the disease. A family history is frequently elicited. Tinnitus may also be present.

Surgery for otosclerosis may restore normal hearing but also carries a small risk of total hearing loss. Use of a hearing aid has no complications, but is often refused (Fig. 3).

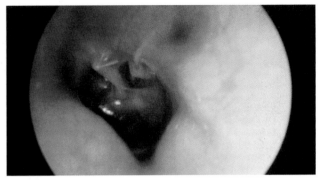

Fig. 1 **Multiple exostoses may lead to narrowing of the external meati.** They are sited at the osseocartilaginous junction of the ear canal.

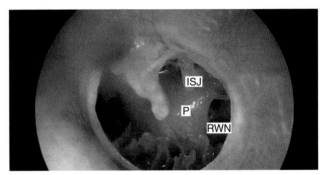

Fig. 2 **A subtotal perforation of the left eardrum.** The round window niche (RWN), the inudostapedial joint (ISJ) and promontory (P) are clearly visible.

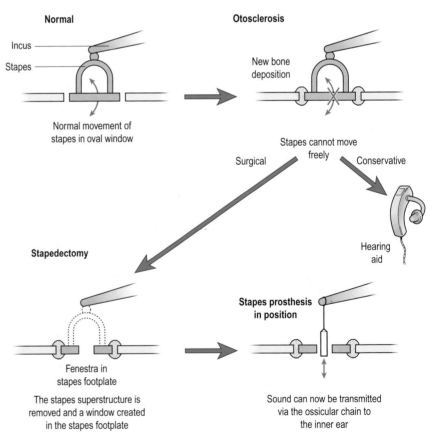

Fig. 3 **The pathology and management of otosclerosis.**

Sensorineural hearing loss

Presbyacusis (common)

Presbyacusis is a progressive loss of hair cells in the cochlea with age. Roughly 1% of cells are lost each year, and this affects the high frequency part of the inner ear first (Fig. 4). It becomes clinically noticeable from the age of about 60–65 years. The degree of loss varies, as does the age of onset. Some patients with presbyacusis have recruitment (reduced dynamic range of hearing) which reduces effective amplification. The threshold for hearing and the uncomfortable level of sound are abnormally close (e.g. 'Speak up, I can't hear you … don't shout so loud!'). Discrimination may also be affected ('I hear you but can't understand you'). There is no treatment to prevent this loss. When a significant social or work handicap is present, a hearing aid may be prescribed. This should be digital so that the pattern of amplification is tailored to the pattern of the individuals hearing loss. Two hearing aids are better than one!

Sudden (idiopathic) hearing loss (rare)

Cochlear failure may occur in a previously normal ear. The patient is suddenly aware of a blockage or rapid deterioration in hearing. Tinnitus or vertigo may be present. The aetiology is thought to be either a virus infection or vascular ischaemia. Treatment is largely empirical, and changes from decade to decade. Currently there is a great deal of interest in the role of steroids and antiviral agents. Preservation of high-frequency hearing on serial audiograms indicates a good prognosis.

Noise exposure (common)

Acoustic trauma occurs from sudden exposure (impact or blast), or from prolonged exposure, e.g. noise of heavy industrial machinery. Levels of 90 dB or greater require ear protection *with properly fitted ear defenders*. After exposure there may be a temporary threshold shift, perceived as 'woolly hearing' and associated with tinnitus. Continued noise exposure will lead to permanent threshold shifts, usually affecting the higher frequencies starting at 4 kHz.

Treatment is by avoidance or employing adequate ear protection in the form of ear defenders. An established hearing loss may benefit from a hearing aid. A system of compensation is available for occupational hearing loss.

Perilymph fistula (rare)

A rupture of the labyrinthine windows (round or oval) will result in leakage of perilymph fluid and a sensorineural type hearing loss. Mild features of imbalance or even frank vertigo may also occur. The rupture is usually preceded by an event that raises the intracranial pressure, e.g. straining to lift. It may also follow a stapedectomy operation where an iatrogenic fistula is sealed but the leak persists. The middle ear should be explored in cases where the hearing is deteriorating; otherwise, there is a risk of total hearing loss. The offending rupture is then sealed with a fat plug.

Inflammatory diseases (rare)

Measles, mumps, meningitis or syphilis may cause cochlear damage and can result in permanent sensorineural hearing loss. Chronic middle ear disease is also often associated with some degree of sensorineural loss.

Ototoxicity

The inner ear has many active metabolic processes which are susceptible to drugs. The cochlea or labyrinth may be affected in isolation or in combination, and this can result in hearing loss and symptoms of imbalance. Agents that are toxic to the renal system commonly affect the ear, e.g. systemic aminoglycosides and cytotoxic agents. Salicylates and quinine have reversible toxicity.

Acoustic tumours

Acoustic tumours are rare, but treatable, tumours of the vestibular element of the eighth cranial nerve. The commonest presentation is a progressive unilateral hearing loss with tinnitus. MRI scanning with gadolinium is the investigation of choice and can demonstrate small tumours (Fig. 5). Current treatment options include serial scanning (for small tumours), surgical excision or stereotactic radiosurgery.

Dysacusis

Despite having normal hearing thresholds, some patients are still unable to hear well, particularly in noisy environments. This is termed dysacusis. The aetiology is presumed to be a cochlear abnormality.

Non-organic hearing loss

Some patients are malingerers, either with a psychological problem or seeking benefits. In such cases the history and serial subjective audiometric tests do not match the clinical observations. Objective assessment obtained with electric response audiometry will unmask any difficult non-organic hearing loss.

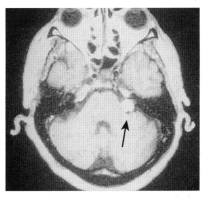

Fig. 5 **An axial view of an acoustic neuroma seen on MRI after injection of gadolinium contrast.** The tumour stands out clearly.

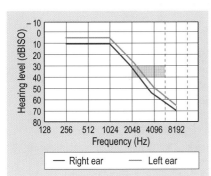

Fig. 4 **A typical audiogram seen in a patient with presbyacusis.** There is a ski-slope-type high-frequency loss. The low frequencies may remain within the normal range.

Hearing loss in adults

- Wax impaction and presbyacusis are the leading causes of hearing loss in adults.
- Most causes of conductive hearing loss are identifiable on otoscopy.
- Otitis media with effusion in adults is rare, so exclude neoplasia of the nasopharynx.
- In otosclerosis the eardrum has a normal appearance.
- A progressive unilateral sensorineural hearing loss should be fully investigated to exclude an acoustic neuroma.

Aids to hearing

Hearing loss is a major disability that can interfere with the social, work and educational spheres of a patient's life. A 35 dB loss in the speech frequencies (500–2000 Hz) can result in major problems. Fortunately, the majority of sufferers may be helped by employing one or more of the remedies available (Table 1).

Table 1 **Aids to hearing**
Electronic aids
Environmental aids
Lipreading/sign language
Cochlear implantation
Organizations for the deaf

Electronic hearing aids

An electronic hearing aid consists of an earpiece, amplifier and a microphone. There is a volume control, and many hearing aids are fitted with a 'T' setting that allows the use of electromagnetic induction waves to provide sound and cut out extraneous background noise.

A variety of aids is shown in Figure 1. The majority of patients will be fitted with a postauricular hearing aid which is relatively unobtrusive. However, severe hearing loss may only be assisted by BW (body worn) aids. It is possible to incorporate the aid into a spectacle frame if desired. Miniaturized aids can also be worn in the ear or inserted into the ear canal.

Fitting aids to both ears is preferable in most patients. It is vital to counsel the patient that discrimination may not necessarily be improved, but that amplification can provide benefit by better recognition of rhythms and phrases.

Problems with electronic hearing aids

To gain the maximum benefit from the aid, it is important to provide patients with training. It is a shock to many to learn that an aid cannot produce normal hearing. Patients with conductive hearing losses have better results with aids than those with sensorineural losses. This is due to the fact that many of the latter losses are associated with a phenomenon called 'recruitment', where loud sounds are heard exceptionally loudly so that the amplification from a hearing aid merely adds to the patient's difficulties.

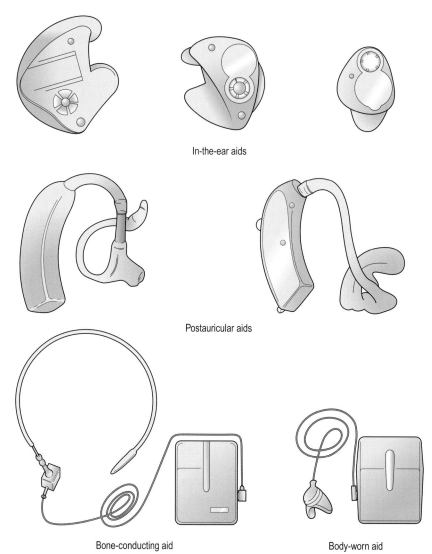

In-the-ear aids

Postauricular aids

Bone-conducting aid

Body-worn aid

Fig. 1 **A selection of hearing aids.** The patient's hearing loss, manual dexterity and vanity will determine the precise aid that is recommended.

The common problems encountered with electronic aids are listed in Table 2. Probably the most frequent difficulty is with acoustic feedback. This produces the familiar high-pitched whistle and is particularly seen in patients who require high amplification, and in whom the ear mould allows sound to escape into the microphone. A similar event will occur if the mould is incorrectly inserted, as is frequently seen in the elderly suffering from arthritic joints.

A persistent otorrhoea may occur due to allergy to the mould. Alternative non-allergenic material can be employed. In some patients this manoeuvre is simply ineffective and, in others, continued insertion of a mould produces otitis externa or a discharge from a mastoid cavity. Such cases may benefit from a bone conducting aid worn as a headband with the microphone abutting firmly onto the mastoid. However, these are cosmetically unsightly.

More recent alternatives are bone conduction aids that are anchored in the temporal bone. The external stimulator sets the aid in vibration either across the intervening skin or by a direct percutaneous attachment

Table 2 **Common problems with electronic hearing aids**	
Problem	**Cause**
Feedback	Badly fitting ear mould
Otorrhoea	Ear infection
	Allergy to mould
No sound	Dead battery
	Blocked tube

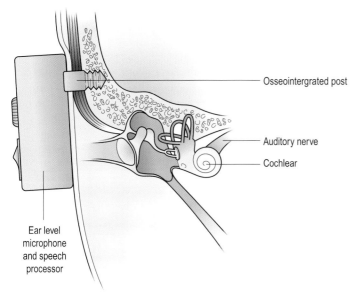

Fig. 2 **Osseointegrated aid.** This avoids many of the problems of traditional aids.

Labels: Osseointergrated post, Auditory nerve, Cochlear, Ear level microphone and speech processor

facility (Fig. 2; Fig. 3, p. 24). Such aids do not suffer the feedback problems of conventional air conduction aids and also have the advantage of greatly reduced background noise.

Environmental aids

There are many products available that may assist the deafened patient in routine daily life. Doorbells may be changed to buzzers or flashing lights. Telephones can be fitted with volume controls and be converted to be used with the 'T' induction aid in a hearing aid.

Lipreading and manual communication

Most patients with hearing loss requiring aiding will benefit from the development of lipreading skills. These are essential in any severe or progressive hearing loss. Special classes are run by most hearing aid departments. A deafened person is better able to lipread if the speaker assists in ensuring certain optimal conditions (Fig. 3).

If at all possible, normal speech and language development in children with severe hearing loss should be encouraged by amplification of any residual hearing. This oral method is preferred to the manual communication skills using sign language, as the latter requires determination and repeated practice to acquire, and can only be used with others who have similar skills.

Cochlear implants

A cochlear implant is a device used in patients with a non-functioning cochlea but who have a normal cochlear nerve. Unaidable bilateral sensorineural deafness is the main criterion for potential implantation. The nerve can be stimulated by placing an electrode into the cochlea (Fig. 4). A processor converts speech into electrical signals that are transmitted to the electrode. The cochlear nerve is stimulated, giving clues to frequencies and cadences. With modern sound processors a severely deafened individual can be trained to communicate with a very high degree of success.

Organizations for the deaf

In the UK there are many local social services and educational organizations to support the deafened person. Three national groups may be contacted for help and advice. These are:

- Royal National Institute for the Deaf (RNID)
- Link, The British Centre for Deafened People
- National Deaf Children's Society (NDCS).

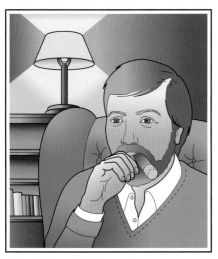

- Poor background lighting
- Sitting in shade
- Covering face and lips with hands
- Speaking with cigarette, cigar or pipe in mouth
- Beard and moustache

Fig. 3 **To assist a deafened person in lipreading, the speaker should avoid all the above.**

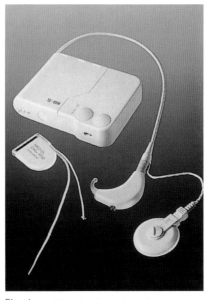

Fig. 4 **Cochlear implantation.** The device is employed to stimulate any residual cochlear nerve fibres via the electrode implanted in the scala tympani of the cochlea.

Aids to hearing

- Hearing aids do not produce normal hearing.
- Only appropriate aids for the patient's hearing loss, correctly used, will provide any benefit.
- Environmental aids are extremely valuable.
- Lipreading should be instituted early rather than late.
- Providing a deaf person with the optimal conditions will enable them to lipread.
- Manual communication is only possible with both parties having the requisite skills.
- Cochlear implants are suitable for only very few patients with bilateral total hearing loss; they cannot reproduce speech.

Otalgia

Otalgia, or earache, is common in both children and adults. Local causes of otalgia are usually diagnosed by examination of the pinna, ear canal and tympanic membrane. If the ear is normal, the pain may be referred by one of several cranial nerves supplying the external and middle ear.

Otological causes of otalgia

Acute otitis externa

Acute otitis externa is common in patients with eczematous ear canal skin, and in those who produce trauma with cotton buds. Moist, humid environments predispose to ear canal infections. Symptoms may vary from itching and irritation to excruciating pain. Streptococci, staphylococci, *Pseudomonas* and fungi are the usual infecting agents. Pressure on the tragus or manipulation of the pinna at its root will cause discomfort. In the early stages the canal is red and tender and there may be a thin discharge. Hearing loss occurs later with oedema of the canal and accumulation of debris.

Treatment is outlined in Figure 1. A very convenient ear dressing is the otowick, which after insertion into the ear canal will expand if topical drops are applied. Discharge should be sent for culture. Relapse is often due to residual debris in the meatus. Prolonged use of antibiotic/steroid drops promotes secondary fungal otitis, e.g. *Aspergillus* (Fig. 2, p. 14). Itching may be controlled by 1% hydrocortisone cream applied with a cotton bud, but only after the infection has been treated.

Furunculosis

Furunculosis is an infection of a hair follicle in the outer ear canal. *Severe* throbbing pain with pyrexia precedes rupture of

the abscess. Examination and drainage under anaesthetic may be required.

Malignant otitis externa

Malignant otitis externa is an aggressive form of otitis externa; the term malignant is a misnomer. The pathophysiology is a spreading osteomyelitis of the temporal bone caused by the organism *Pseudomonas pyocyaneus*. It tends to occur in immunocompromised patients, such as elderly diabetics. Marked granulations are formed in the ear canal. The infection spreads to involve the middle ear and the lower cranial nerves.

CT and isotope scanning provide information on the extent of the osteomyelitis (Fig. 2). Treatment comprises local aural toilet and insertion of wicks impregnated with an antipseudomonal accompanied by high-dose antibiotics. Surgery for debridement may be necessary in patients in whom the disease progresses despite conservative treatment.

Myringitis bullosa

Myringitis bullosa is a localized form of otitis externa where blisters form on the eardrum and deep meatus. It presents as an excruciating earache and is presumed to be a viral infection. Treatment is symptomatic.

Perichondritis

Perichondritis can follow severe otitis externa, or be subsequent to trauma. The infected cartilage produces a swollen red and tender pinna. Oedema may spread onto the face and the pretragal lymph nodes are enlarged. Local astringents (e.g. magnesium sulphate) and systemic antibiotics are required to prevent permanent damage to the cartilage and an ugly cosmetic appendage.

Acute otitis media

Acute otitis media is a common cause of severe otalgia in children. Inflammation of the middle ear cleft usually follows an upper respiratory tract infection which ascends via the Eustachian tube. The eardrum

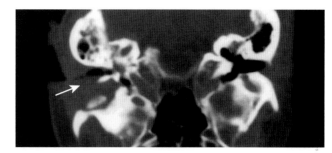

Fig. 2 **A case of malignant otitis externa showing extensive destruction of the temporal bone.** The facial nerve is frequently affected, but the other lower cranial nerves (glossopharyngeal, vagus and hypoglossal) become involved as the osteomyelitis spreads.

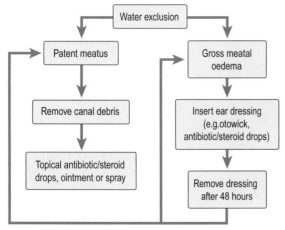

Fig. 1 **Treatment of acute otitis externa.** Systemic treatment involves the use of oral analgesics and antibiotics.

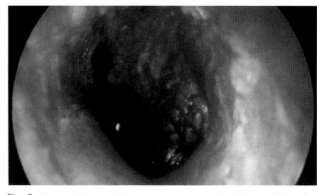

Fig. 3 **Acute otitis media is a common cause of otalgia in children.** If allowed to progress, the initial infection of the eardrum leads to bulging as the middle ear pressure increases due to pus formation, with the ultimate rupture of the drum.

becomes retracted as the tube is blocked, and an inflammatory middle ear exudate develops. Pressure in the middle ear produces severe pain, and the eardrum becomes congested and bulging (Fig. 3). At this stage the patient is quite unwell, with fever and tachycardia. Eardrum rupture may then occur, producing a bloodstained discharge with relief of the pain.

Antibiotic treatment of acute otitis media is somewhat controversial as many cases are of viral origin. After 24–48 hours, if spontaneous resolution has not occurred, a broad-spectrum antibiotic to cover *Haemophilus* and Streptococci is indicated. Prior to this, analgesics and nasal decongestants may be employed. The discharging ear should be swabbed, mopped and kept dry. Resolution is usual, but a middle ear effusion may persist. It is not uncommon for hearing to remain muffled for up to 1 month or more in adults. Children frequently suffer more than one attack of acute otitis media. If this is associated with persisting middle ear effusions, then myringotomy and grommet insertion, possibly with adenoidectomy, may be indicated. An alternative is to give a low dose of antibiotic, e.g. 125 mg penicillin, at night for 6 weeks. Acute otitis media accompanying childhood infections, e.g. measles, may be so severe that the eardrum fails to heal, leaving a large central perforation.

The complications of otitis media usually arise from inadequate treatment or non-compliance. Inflammation of the mastoid air cell system often occurs with acute otitis media, and is controlled with antibiotics. However, suppuration in the mastoid (acute mastoiditis) is serious and potentially life-threatening (Fig. 1, p. 16).

Acute otitic barotrauma
Acute otitic barotrauma may occur during descent in aircraft. It leads to severe otalgia and occasionally rupture of the eardrum with a bloody otorrhoea.

Herpes zoster oticus (Ramsay Hunt syndrome)
The facial nerve ganglion may be affected by shingles. This produces severe pain, with vesicles in the ear canal and on the concha, and is frequently accompanied by facial palsy (Fig. 3, p. 19). Administration of antivirals such as famciclovir or aciclovir, if the vesicles are recognized early, may prevent permanent damage to the facial nerve.

Neoplasia of the ear
Otalgia in these patients is caused by perichondritis or nerve involvement by tumour (p. 114).

Non-otological causes of otalgia

The ear has a rich sensory supply from several cranial nerves (trigeminal, glossopharyngeal and vagus) and the posterior roots of the 2nd and 3rd cervical nerves. If examination of the pinna, ear canal and eardrum is normal, otalgia is a *referred* pain. It is important, therefore, to examine the peripheral areas innervated by these nerves (Fig. 4).

Referred otalgia in children
Tonsillitis with otalgia is frequently seen in young children. Referred otalgia is common 5–7 days after tonsillectomy. However, the ear should be examined to exclude an acute otitis media. Dental disease is also a common cause of referred otalgia in children. Diets high in sugar content have led to a prevalence of tooth decay. Teething, particularly if unerupted, may cause referred pain. Upper respiratory tract infections are also commonly associated with otalgia due to Eustachian tube dysfunction.

Referred otalgia in adults
Dental pathology is a common cause of referred otalgia. Impacted molars may result in local pain and referred otalgia.

Anatomical and functional abnormalities of the temporomandibular joint (TMJ) are a frequent cause of referred earache. Spasm of the joint muscles may also produce earache, which is aggravated by dental abnormalities, e.g. malocclusion, tilting and loss of teeth. The joint is usually tender to palpation, particularly during jaw opening. Management is directed at relieving any muscle spasm and correcting dental abnormalities.

Cervical spondylosis can cause referred otalgia in the elderly. There is general tenderness around and behind the ear. The range of neck movements, although restricted, may reproduce the earache. Treatment is physiotherapy and anti-inflammatory and analgesic medication.

It is vital not to miss neoplastic causes of referred otalgia. A cancer in the upper air and food passages may be a cause. All sites should be inspected and the neck palpated for masses.

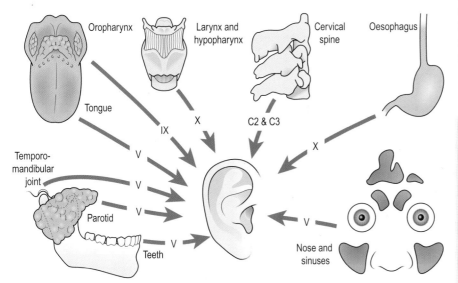

Fig. 4 **Referred or non-otological otalgia.** This can be due to pathology in those sites which have a dual nerve supply with the ear. All these potential peripheral areas must be examined in all cases of referred otalgia.

Otalgia

- Otalgia may be due to otological or non-otological causes. If the ear is normal, look at distant sites.

- In children, acute otitis media, otitis media with effusion and a negative middle ear pressure are the most frequent otological causes of otalgia.

- In adults the temporomandibular joint and cervical spine are common sites of referred otalgia.

- Never forget neoplasms of the upper aerodigestive tract as a cause of referred otalgia in adults.

Otorrhoea

Otorrhoea – an aural discharge – may arise from diseases of the ear canal, but is more commonly associated with middle ear infections. Patients with otorrhoea usually have a degree of hearing loss (p. 6) but may experience no pain. Soft wax can be mistaken for a discharge, but, at the other extreme, daily offensive otorrhoea may be ignored by some patients with a serious underlying middle ear disease. The character of the discharge provides clues to the aetiology (Table 1).

Otorrhoea from ear canal disease

Acute otitis externa

Acute infection of the external ear canal has already been discussed (p. 12). Although otalgia is the predominant symptom, some degree of otorrhoea is common (Fig. 1). It is not unusual for certain general skin conditions to cause otitis externa with otorrhoea, e.g. psoriasis, seborrhoeic dermatitis and eczema. It is useful to emphasize that early relapse after treatment with eardrops is usually due to inadequate aural toilet, or colonization of the canal by a secondary fungal growth (Fig. 2). Treatment of any underlying eczema in the canal, e.g. with 1% hydrocortisone cream is important when the inflammation has settled.

Chronic otitis externa

Chronic otitis externa is usually bilateral, painless and tends to relapse. The skin of the canal is permanently thickened and easily traumatized. All canal debris should be removed and the skin kept dry. Antibiotic drops are not advised unless there is acute inflammation. Indeed, they may precipitate an allergic reaction or predispose to fungal infection.

Furunculosis

Furunculosis (p. 12), a severe form of acute otitis externa, produces persistent throbbing pain and a seropurulent otorrhoea if the abscess ruptures. The patient may require an anaesthetic for examination and drainage. Treatment is then continued as for acute otitis externa.

Otorrhoea from middle ear disease

There are two main types of chronic otitis media. Both produce otorrhoea and hearing loss, and are invariably associated with a defect of the eardrum. One is a mucosal disease; the other causes bone loss and may cause serious complications. Otalgia is infrequent.

Chronic suppurative otitis media (tubotympanic disease)

Rupture of the tympanic membrane in acute otitis media produces a bloodstained, mucopurulent otorrhoea. The eardrum usually heals quickly, but if the inflammation persists and the eardrum skin fails to heal over the margins of the rupture, a persistent perforation will result. Persistent or recurrent mucoid discharge may then occur, especially if water enters the middle ear or in episodes of upper respiratory tract infections. Perforations as a result of recurrent acute otitis media usually occur in the pars tensa and do not involve the anulus. They are rarely associated with serious disease and are referred to as 'safe' perforations (Figs 3 & 4).

The initial treatment of a discharging perforation is aural toilet combined with topical steroid

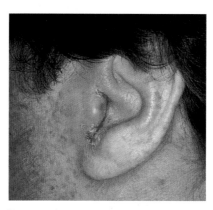

Fig. 1 **Acute otitis externa.** The ear canal is occluded due to gross swelling. Manipulation of the pinna or tragus is painful, and chewing commonly produces discomfort due to the temporomandibular joint causing movement of the cartilaginous portion of the external ear canal.

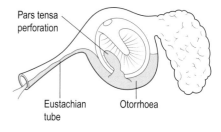

- Infection in lower part of middle ear cavity
- Not usually involving the mastoid

Fig. 3 **Chronic suppurative otitis media (tubotympanic disease).** This is associated with a central perforation of the pars tensa. The otorrhoea is usually profuse and mucoid in the active infection, and exacerbated by any dysfunction of the Eustachian tube, e.g. acute rhinitis.

Table 1 **Characteristics of otorrhoea in relation to aetiology**	
Character of otorrhoea	**Potential aetiology**
Watery	Eczema of the ear canal, cerebrospinal fluid (rare)
Purulent	Acute otitis externa, furunculosis
Mucoid*	Chronic suppurative otitis media (tubotympanic) with a perforation
Mucopurulent/ bloody	Trauma, acute otitis media, carcinoma of the ear (rare)
Foul smelling	Chronic suppurative otitis media (atticoantral) with cholesteatoma

*Mucous glands are located only in the middle ear.

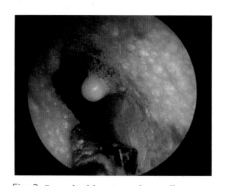

Fig. 2 **Fungal otitis externa is usually caused by candidial or aspergillus species.** This illustration shows the tiny black spores seen in infection with *Aspergillus niger*.

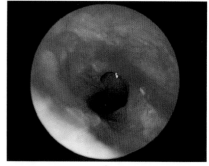

Fig. 4 **A central perforation involving the pars tensa associated with chronic suppurative otitis media.** This shows an infected perforation with mucoid discharge in the external ear canal.

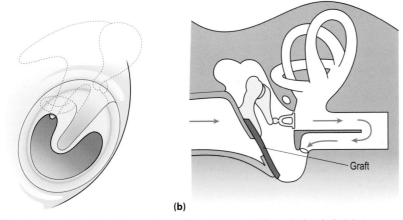

(a)   (b)

Fig. 5 **A simple perforation of the eardrum with an intact mobile ossicular chain (a).** An underlay graft to repair the perforation **(b)**.

eardrops. This will dry up most discharging ears so that an accurate assessment can be made of the drum head and middle ear mucosa. If the perforation persists, the patient has chronic suppurative otitis media (tubotympanic type), which may be inactive or active (if discharging). Use of antibiotic eardrops is no longer recommended routinely as many contain ototoxic aminoglycosides. Some eye drops, such as those containing ofloxacin or ciprofloxacin, are not ototoxic and are effective; however, they are not currently licensed in the UK for aural use.

For those patients who have little trouble, a hearing aid to overcome hearing difficulties may be all that is required. Surgery is recommended for recurring discharge, for patients who are regular swimmers, and to produce a hearing improvement. The material for a graft is usually the patient's own temporalis fascia, which is easily accessible (Fig. 5).

Chronic suppurative otitis media (atticoantral disease)

Long-standing Eustachian tube dysfunction may produce retractions and perforations of the tympanic membrane in the attic region, or may involve the anulus (Figs 6 & 7). These are associated with *cholesteatoma* (keratinizing epithelium in the middle ear). This is a destructive disease and can be life-threatening due to the potential complications.

Aural discharge may be scanty, but is offensive because of underlying osteitis. Bone destruction may occur towards the middle or posterior cranial fossae, often unrecognized until an intracranial complication occurs. The hearing loss with atticoantral disease is usually marked.

Because of the dangerous nature of this disease, surgery is invariably recommended. Excision of disease with preservation of hearing involves surgery on the mastoid and middle ear (mastoidectomy; p. 16). Usually the mastoid is exteriorized by removing the posterior ear canal wall to produce a cavity that can be inspected from the ear canal and cleaned as required. The

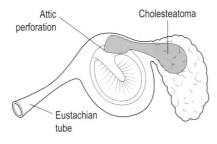

- Infection in upper part of middle ear cavity — usually involving the mastoid
- Often associated with cholesteatoma

Fig. 6 **Chronic suppurative otitis media (atticoantral disease).** This is associated with a marginal perforation, often in the attic region (pars flaccida). The otorrhoea is usually scanty and foul smelling.

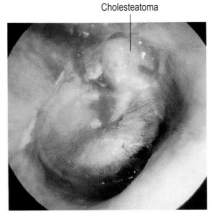

Fig. 7 **Chronic suppurative otitis media of the atticoantral variety, seen in the attic.** Discharge and white keratin debris are seen in the attic perforation.

drum defect may be grafted to minimize postoperative mucous discharge and optimize the hearing.

Discharging mastoid cavities

Many patients have either persistent or recurrent otorrhoea from surgically created mastoid cavities. There are many causes for this and most are amenable to treatment (Table 2). Uncontrolled infection of the middle ear or mastoid cavities may over many years predispose to carcinoma. This rare complication is heralded by a change in character of the otorrhoea from mucopurulent to bloody. It is invariably accompanied by the development of progressive otalgia and a facial paralysis.

Fracture of the temporal bone

A severe blow to the temporal or parietal region may result in a fracture of the temporal bone (p. 42). A conductive hearing loss is due to a combination of blood in the middle ear, ossicular disruption and tympanic membrane perforation. Sensorineural hearing loss will result if the fracture passes through the cochlea. Cerebrospinal fluid otorrhoea may occur but usually settles spontaneously. The patient should be prescribed systemic antibiotics.

Table 2 **Causes and treatment of persistently discharging mastoid cavities**	
Cause	**Treatment**
Small external opening	Enlarge meatus
Infection	Local toilet and topical antibiotic/steroid drops
Residual cholesteatoma	Revision mastoid surgery
Allergy to topical drops	Discontinue drops
High posterior canal wall	Surgery to lower canal wall
Neoplasia	Surgery ± radiotherapy

Otorrhoea

- Carefully examine an aural discharge; its appearance and odour may lead to a diagnosis.

- The integrity of the eardrum must be assessed in patients with otorrhoea.

- Conservative treatment with local aural toilet and topical antibiotics is effective in tubotympanic chronic suppurative otitis media.

- Mastoid surgery will be required in cases of atticoantral chronic suppurative otitis media (cholesteatoma).

- Beware of a change in the character of a chronically discharging ear, particularly if accompanied by otalgia. It may herald development of neoplasia.

Complications of middle ear infections

Ready access to medical treatment and the use of antibiotics has reduced the incidence of complications from acute otitis media. Mastoiditis is probably the most common complication and is more frequent in children. However,

Table 1 Complications of middle ear infections	
Type	**Complication**
Extracranial	Acute mastoiditis
	Facial paralysis
	Labyrinthitis
Intracranial	Meningitis
	Abscess
	— extradural
	— subdural
	— temporal
	— cerebellar
	Lateral sinus thrombosis

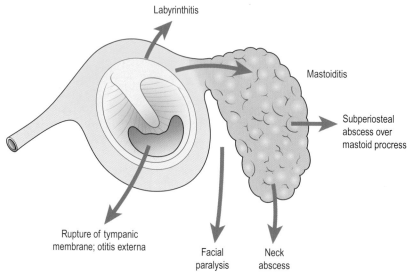

Fig. 1 **Extracranial complications of middle ear infection.**

chronic ear disease is still responsible for cases of intracranial suppuration, which can be life threatening. It is useful to classify complications of middle ear disease into extracranial and intracranial (Table 1).

Extracranial complications

Acute mastoiditis
Mastoiditis is preceded by acute otitis media and is usually seen in young children. Inflammation of the mastoid lining produces severe pain – usually localized over the mastoid process. Perforation of the eardrum from otitis media may relieve the initial discomfort, but a gradual increase in pain with tachycardia and pyrexia suggests extension into the mastoid (Fig. 1). Early physical signs include a sagging or oedematous posterior ear canal wall, with oedema over the mastoid and zygomatic areas. Eventually the pinna is pushed down and out by a subperiosteal abscess (Fig. 2), and the drum head bulges or discharges pus.

Inadequate medical treatment may allow development of mastoiditis from acute otitis media, but some cases progress so rapidly as to present with mastoiditis.

In the early stages, administration of intravenous antibiotics may produce resolution of the inflammation. Prolonged treatment is necessary to ensure that resolution is complete and the hearing returns to normal. If there is any doubt about improvement, or if a subperiosteal abscess has developed, a cortical mastoidectomy is performed (Fig. 3).

Facial paralysis
If there is a dehiscence in the bony covering of the facial nerve in the middle ear, an acute inflammation may cause a temporary paralysis

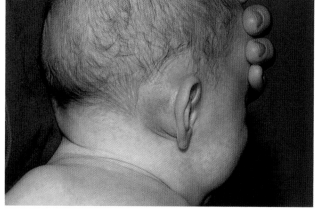

Fig. 2 **A child with acute otitis media which has progressed to acute mastoiditis, with development of a subperiosteal abscess.** Notice the absence of the postauricular sulcus and how the pinna is pushed down and outward.

which recovers as the infection subsides. Exploration of the ear and mastoid is indicated if there is pre-existing chronic ear disease involving the nerve.

Labyrinthitis
Labyrinthitis may occur from acute or chronic ear disease. Signs of labyrinthine inflammation include giddiness and loss of balance with nausea and vomiting. Hearing loss is sensorineural. The patient lies still in bed with the affected ear uppermost (this reduces the sensation of giddiness). High-dose parenteral antibiotics are given to arrest the infection and prevent meningitis. Surgery may be required in cases with pus formation.

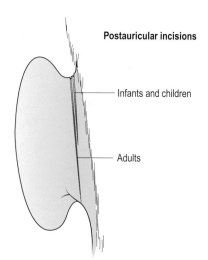

Fig. 3 **Surgical approach to the mastoid air system.** This can be made through a postauricular incision. In children, the incision is not extended inferiorly due to the risk of damaging the facial nerve, as the mastoid tip which protects it is underdeveloped.

Intracranial complications

Meningitis

Meningitis may occur from infection via the labyrinth, the lateral sinus or through direct extension from the middle ear. Pneumococcal meningitis commonly occurs from the ear. Initially the patient is pyrexial with a headache; later, confusion, irritability and neck stiffness occur. Diagnosis is by lumbar puncture, but a CT scan may be indicated to exclude an intracranial abscess. Intravenous antibiotics should initially control the infection before any surgery is contemplated. Recurrent bacterial meningitis requires an ENT assessment of the ear and paranasal sinuses for foci of infection, or for evidence of a CSF leak.

Intracranial abscess

The development of an intracranial abscess (Fig. 4) carries a significant mortality. An extradural abscess in the middle or posterior cranial fossa can occur by direct extension of middle ear infection. Erosion of the dural plate produces a dural reaction with granulation and abscess formation.

Temporal lobe abscess

A temporal lobe abscess may complicate acute or chronic middle ear disease (Fig. 5). The patient has a history of hearing loss and/or otorrhoea, and develops signs of cerebritis (headache, rigors, fever and vomiting). There may follow a latent period of up to several weeks, during which time the ear disease may appear to be controlled. The patient may then present with signs of raised intracranial pressure or focal signs of an abscess, e.g. a fit, paralysis or visual field changes. Patients with these signs require a CT or MRI scan. In all cases of cerebritis, high-dose parenteral antibiotics are required. Drainage of an established abscess is usually via a burr hole, and repeated aspiration of the cavity may be necessary.

Cerebellar abscess

A cerebellar abscess is uncommon, but can present with or after treatment for mastoiditis. Homolateral cerebellar signs of nystagmus, past pointing and ataxia, together with headache, demand an urgent CT scan (Fig. 6) and surgical drainage.

Thrombosis of the lateral venous sinus

Thrombosis of the lateral venous sinus occurs from extension of suppuration within the mastoid. Clot builds up within the vessel until the lumen is occluded. The patient may develop rigors and a high fever, but these signs can be masked by previous antibiotics. The diagnosis is often made at mastoidectomy.

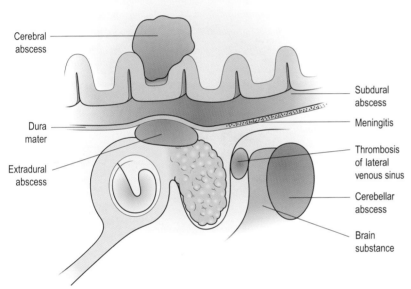

Fig. 4 **Intracranial complications of middle ear infection.**

Labels: Cerebral abscess, Dura mater, Extradural abscess, Subdural abscess, Meningitis, Thrombosis of lateral venous sinus, Cerebellar abscess, Brain substance

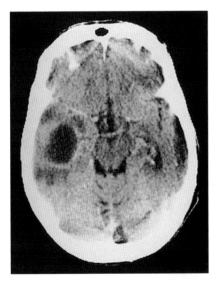

Fig. 5 **Temporal lobe abscess.** This can result from extension of middle ear disease superiorly through the roof of the middle ear cavity (tegmen tympani).

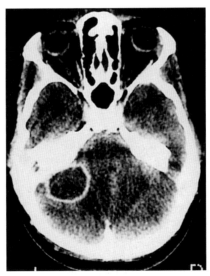

Fig. 6 **Cerebellar abscess seen on CT scan.**

Complications of middle ear infections

- Acute mastoiditis is the commonest complication of acute middle ear infection.
- All patients with intracranial inflammation should have an otoscopic examination.
- Intracranial complications can occur without otological symptoms.
- Treatment of intracranial complications takes precedence over therapy for underlying middle ear infection.
- CT or MRI provide fast, accurate and non-invasive techniques for diagnosing intracranial complications.

Facial palsy

The facial nerve has a complex course from the brain stem through the temporal bone and the parotid gland, before innervating the muscles of facial expression (Fig. 1). Running alongside this motor nerve are sensory fibres conveying taste from the anterior part of the tongue, and secretomotor fibres destined for the lacrimal, submandibular and sublingual glands.

Damage to the facial nerve results in facial weakness and a considerable cosmetic deformity (Fig. 2). The neurological level of damage determines the clinical picture. In supranuclear lesions, e.g. stroke, the forehead is often spared due to bilateral innervation. Infranuclear lesions produce a lower motor neurone paralysis with both the upper and lower facial muscles involved.

The degree of recovery is dependent on the extent of nerve damage. A reversible conduction block (neurapraxia) results from minor injury to the nerve. Complete recovery is usual within 6 weeks.

More severe lesions cause axon degeneration, and recovery occurs by regeneration. This may take from 3 to 12 months, and recovery is rarely complete. The commoner causes of facial paralysis are shown in Table 1.

Clinical history

A detailed history may reveal the likely aetiology of a facial paralysis and also its site. For example, Bell's palsy and herpes zoster oticus (Ramsay Hunt syndrome; Fig. 3) are frequently heralded by otalgia before the onset of facial weakness. A chronically discharging ear complicated by facial nerve deficits is invariably due to the atticoantral (cholesteatoma) type of chronic suppurative otitis media. Facial paralysis resulting from surgical

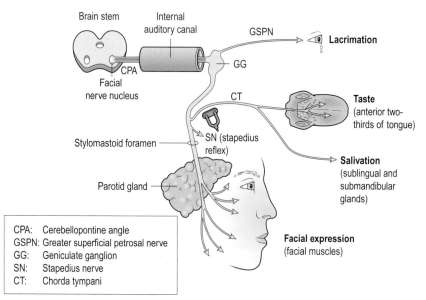

Fig. 1 **Topography of the facial nerve.**

CPA:	Cerebellopontine angle
GSPN:	Greater superficial petrosal nerve
GG:	Geniculate ganglion
SN:	Stapedius nerve
CT:	Chorda tympani

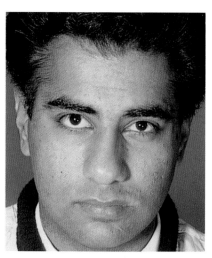

'**Relax**' Note slightly wider palpebral fissure on right eye

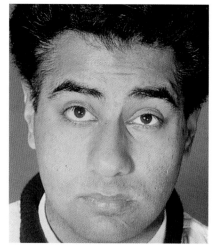

'**Raise eyebrows**' Note reduced furrowing of forehead on right

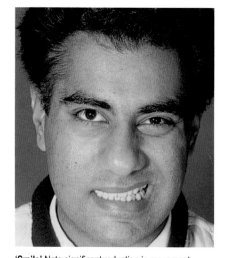

'**Smile**' Note significant reduction in movement on right, giving a wry look to the mouth

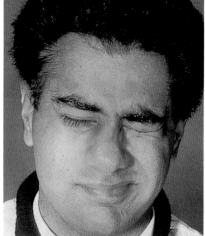

'**Close eyes tight**' Note obvious weakness on the right

Fig. 2 **A patient with right-sided facial paralysis.** Notice the cosmetic deformity on facial movement.

Table 1 **Causes of facial palsy**	
Site	**Aetiology**
Intracranial	Acoustic neuroma
	CVA*
	Brain stem tumour*
Intratemporal	Bell's palsy
	Herpes zoster oticus
	Middle ear infection
	Trauma
	— surgical
	— temporal bone fracture
Extratemporal	Parotid tumours
Miscellaneous	Sarcoidosis, polyneuritis

*Supranuclear lesions.

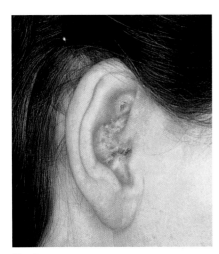

Fig. 3 **A florid case of herpes zoster oticus (Ramsay Hunt syndrome).** The vesicles are clearly visible in the concha. A partial facial paralysis was also present.

trauma (particularly in otological procedures) and temporal bone fractures is easily diagnosed. Tissue masses in the region of the parotid, with associated facial paralysis, indicate malignancy. However, the sinister malignant adenoid cystic carcinoma of the parotid may present with an isolated cosmetic facial defect and no obvious palpable neck mass.

Enquiries should be made about alteration in taste, which if present implies the lesion is above the chorda tympani. A sensitivity to high-intensity sound (hyperacusis) indicates a lesion above the stapedius nerve, with a resultant absence of the stapedius reflex. A dry eye due to reduced lacrimation suggests pathology at, or proximal to, the geniculate ganglion.

Clinical examination

It is important to establish whether the facial paralysis is supranuclear (forehead spared) or infranuclear (Fig. 4). Most patients fear a stroke as the cause, and this can be excluded rapidly if the frontalis muscle is paretic. The facial movements should be assessed in the forehead, around the eyes, the cheek and mouth. Otoscopic examination may reveal the vesicles of herpes zoster oticus, or the presence of cholesteatoma in a chronically discharging ear. Rarely, a glomus jugulare tumour may be visible. A parotid tumour may be palpable in the neck, but examination of the oropharynx is essential to exclude a lesion of the deep lobe of the parotid, pushing the tonsil medially. A complete examination of the cranial nerve should be made. Further investigations may include hearing tests, particularly if otoscopy was normal.

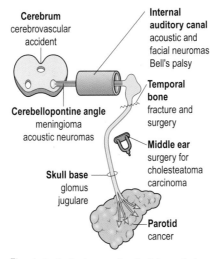

Fig. 4 **Pathologies causing facial paralysis.**

Rarely, an acoustic neuroma or facial nerve tumour may present as an isolated facial paralysis. Electrodiagnostic tests may also assist in assessing the type of nerve damage (neurapraxia, etc.) and give some indication as to the prognosis.

Management

Management of facial paralysis is dependent on the aetiology; the psychological effects are great so the cosmetic defect should be alleviated and the facial nerve provided with the milieu for recovery.

In an established palsy, an ophthalmological opinion should be sought. The patient's eye should be carefully examined to ensure that the cornea is covered by the upper lid during eye closure (Bell's sign). This reduces the risk of corneal abrasion, but other prophylactic measures should be instituted.

These might include:

- regular use of eyedrops or silicone ointment
- spectacles with a side protector
- insertion of gold weights in the upper eyelid
- surgical procedures such as canthoplasty, lower lid augmentation, etc.

Facial cosmesis may be improved by muscle transfer in established palsy or hypoglossal–facial anastomosis. A deep-plane facelift can also be helpful.

Complete nerve section may follow temporal bone fractures, and some otological procedures result in total paralysis. Such cases require either end-to-end anastomosis or insertion of a nerve graft after excision of the damaged portion of the facial nerve.

In partial paralysis, e.g. after ear surgery, the simple act of removing any packing may alleviate nerve compression and allow recovery.

Specific causes of facial palsy

Bell's palsy (idiopathic facial paralysis)

Bell's palsy is the commonest cause of facial paralysis and is a diagnosis of exclusion. The presumed aetiology is inflammation of the facial nerve which leads to compression within the bony canal, causing a conduction block. Current thinking is that many of these cases may be due to Herpes simplex type 1. Discomfort or pain around the mastoid may precede the palsy. Loss of hearing, taste and occasionally hyperacusis can also be present. When the palsy remains incomplete, almost all patients have a satisfactory recovery, usually commencing within 3 weeks of onset. Recovery rates are less good when the palsy is complete: about 85% of patients have an excellent outcome, 10% a partial recovery and 5% a poor outcome. Steroids may be prescribed to reduce the inflammatory swelling of the nerve, although there is no hard evidence that they affect outcome. Similarly, antivirals are commonly administered but, again, hard evidence is lacking.

Trauma

Trauma may cause damage to the facial nerve within the temporal bone or peripherally in the facial soft tissues. Lacerations anterior or inferior to the tragus may divide branches lying in the parotid gland.

Facial palsy

- Many patients equate facial palsy with having suffered a stroke.

- If the forehead is involved, the palsy is due to an infranuclear (lower motor neurone) lesion and reassurance can be given that a CVA has not occurred.

- Always perform otoscopy in cases of facial palsy, as it may reveal the few treatable causes of facial paralysis.

- Bell's palsy is a diagnosis of exclusion.

- A Bell's palsy which is complete or which shows no evidence of recovery within 6 weeks requires referral to an ENT surgeon.

- Parotid neoplasia may present as a facial palsy.

- Patients undergoing mastoid surgery should be counselled on the risks of facial nerve damage.

- The major complications of a facial palsy are related to the eye and to self-image.

Disorders of balance — Introduction and otological causes

Imbalance, dizziness or 'vertigo' can all be symptoms of an underlying disturbance of the vestibular system (p. 2). The pathology may be peripheral (otological) or central (brain stem), producing an illusion of movement (vertigo). There are many inputs into the vestibular system – eyes, ears, joint proprioception, signals from the cerebellum (Fig. 1). Each of these inputs may influence balance, as will primary disorders of the labyrinths and their central connections.

Symptoms

History taking is the key to diagnosing balance disorders. It is important to characterize the main symptom. Patients tend to use the term 'dizzy' to describe a variety of different symptoms. In general, the symptoms may be classified as in Table 1.

It is important to question the patient on the following points:

- the first attack – mode of onset and duration
- changes in hearing and the presence of tinnitus
- relation to activity (head movements, body posture, turning in bed)
- effect of darkness or closing the eyes
- concomitant cardiovascular disease
- drug history (antihypertensives, aminoglycosides)
- alcohol consumption
- anxiety.

The duration of symptoms is important to ascertain, as this is a guide to the potential aetiology (Table 2).

Otological causes of imbalance tend to improve with time due to central compensation, and the symptoms are usually controlled with vestibular sedatives. Non-otological aetiologies of imbalance do not have these features. For example, loss of consciousness or blackout is not a feature of ear disease, but is usually caused by epilepsy or cardiac arrhythmias.

Signs

The tympanic membranes should be examined for evidence of middle ear disease. The eyes are tested for nystagmus (p. 5), which is classified according to the quick phase of the movement.

All the cranial nerve and cerebellar functions are formally assessed. The patient is requested to stand to perform Romberg's test (Fig. 2). An abnormality of gait may be unmasked when the subject walks across the room and turns round. A positional test is mandatory, as are

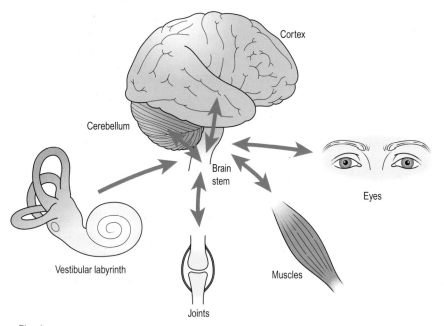

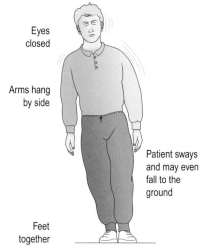

Fig. 2 **The Romberg test.** Sensory input from the eyes is blocked. This may cause swaying or falling in patients with either loss of joint proprioception or peripheral vestibular disturbance.

Fig. 1 **Maintenance of balance.** Balance can only be maintained if the various sensory inputs do not contradict each other. For example, a feeling of dysequilibrium can ensue if the head is suddenly stopped from spinning round. This is due to the vestibular labyrinth still indicating movement of the head while the eyes indicate the head is stationary.

Table 1 **Imbalance: terminology and aetiology**

Term	Symptom	Causes
Vertigo	An illusion of rotary movement, worse in the dark	Peripheral vestibular disease, rarely central vestibular pathology
Lightheadedness	A feeling of fainting	Cardiovascular (postural hypotension, antihypertensives), ototoxic drugs Psychiatric conditions
Unsteadiness	Difficulty with gait, a tendency to fall or veer to one side	Ageing process with general incoordination, rarely neurological
Loss of consciousness, blackouts	Usually a clear-cut history	Neurological (epilepsy), cardiac arrhythmias

Table 2 **Duration of symptoms of imbalance in relation to aetiology**

Duration	Aetiology
Seconds	Cervical spondylosis Postural hypotension Benign paroxysmal positional vertigo
Minutes to hours	Ménière's disease Labyrinthitis
Hours to days	Acute labyrinthine failure (without compensation) Ototoxicity Central vestibular disease

lying and standing blood pressure readings.

General management of acute vertigo

In a severe attack of vertigo, management consists of excluding any serious aetiology and providing support to relieve the symptoms. Patients with associated cardiovascular, neurological or otological signs should be referred on. Reassurance and bed rest are essential. Vestibular sedatives may be required, but can be difficult to administer due to nausea and vomiting. Intramuscular, buccal or suppository preparations can be employed.

After the acute stage, the patient may require intermittent long-term sedatives and is frequently helped by graded head, body and eye exercises. These are designed to enhance the process of central compensation.

Otological causes of imbalance

Figure 3 shows the common otological diseases producing vertigo.

Middle ear disease

- *Otitis media with effusion* (glue ear) often causes children to become unsteady on their feet. If surgery is required, myringotomy, aspiration of fluid and grommet insertion restores stability.
- *Acute otitis media* may produce various symptoms of imbalance, including true vertigo. Treatment is bed rest, antibiotics, analgesics and vestibular sedatives.
- *Chronic suppurative otitis media* (atticoantral disease). Erosive cholesteatoma may invade the labyrinth, producing a fistula connecting the middle and inner ear, which may give a positive fistula sign

(p. 5). Patients with a discharging ear and vertigo should be seen urgently by an ENT surgeon.

Trauma

Stapedectomy operations for otosclerosis where the inner ear is opened may result in vertigo. Vertigo can develop at any stage after stapedectomy and usually results from a perilymph leak around the piston. Temporal bone fractures may involve the labyrinth, causing severe vertigo and nystagmus and can be accompanied by facial nerve paralysis.

Benign paroxysmal positional vertigo

This is an episodic vertigo, usually dramatically described as occurring on turning the head. It can follow an upper respiratory tract infection or head injury. The vertigo lasts several seconds and fatigues with repetitive stimulation such as repeated positional testing (p. 5). Most cases settle spontaneously or with specific physiotherapy manoeuvres. Vestibular sedatives have no therapeutic advantage.

Ménière's disease (endolymphatic hydrops)

Ménière's disease typically affects young to middle-aged adults. The cardinal features are shown in Table 3. Attacks tend to occur in clusters. Distortion of hearing is very characteristic. Acute attacks are very distressing and can lead to chronic unsteadiness.

In the early stages, medical management usually suffices. Reassurance and a reduction in smoking, caffeine and salt intake are felt to be useful. Betahistine (a vasodilator) and diuretics are often prescribed to reduce the endolymphatic fluid imbalance in the

Table 3 **Cardinal features of Ménière's disease**	
Symptom (episodic attacks)	**Descriptive details**
Vertigo	The patient is normal between attacks
Hearing loss	Unilateral or bilateral, but level fluctuates
Tinnitus	Usually precedes an attack of vertigo
Aural fullness	Described as a pressure, fullness or warm feeling in the ear

inner ear. Surgical options include decompressing the inner ear (draining the endolymphatic sac), disconnecting the labyrinth (vestibular neurectomy) or labyrinthectomy (destruction of the labyrinth).

Labyrinthitis/Acute Balance Disorder

When an infection is localized to the vestibular labyrinth, the patient experiences rapid onset of vertigo with the presence of nystagmus. Hearing loss is a feature if the cochlea is involved. The patient may be very unwell for the first 24 hours, but improves as central compensation occurs. True vertigo persisting longer than 36 hours suggests central involvement. Rehabilitation after labyrinthitis can be improved by graduated vestibular exercises. Older people take longer to compensate. Failure of both labyrinths produces a bobbing oscillopsia where the normal control of the eyes is lost. The world shakes up and down as the patient walks.

Other otological causes

Otosclerosis, syphilis and ototoxic drugs (aminoglycosides) can all produce imbalance due to involvement of the labyrinth. Acoustic neuromas may result in a sense of imbalance.

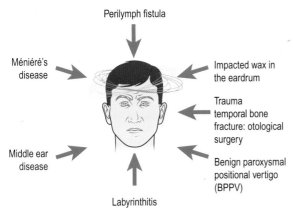

Fig. 3 **Otological causes of imbalance.** The subjective symptom is vertigo which patients may describe as either the environment or themselves spinning. It is obviously an hallucination of movement.

Disorders of balance – Introduction and otological causes

- Ascertain the precise nature of the imbalance.
- The duration of symptoms gives vital clues to the aetiology.
- All patients with vertigo should have an otoscopic examination to exclude middle ear pathology
- All patients should have their hearing assessed to exclude a unilateral deficit and the presence of an acoustic neuroma.
- Otological causes of imbalance improve with time due to central compensation.

Disorders of balance — Non-otological causes

Non-otological diseases producing imbalance are summarized in Figure 1. True vertigo – illusion of rotary movement – is not a feature of non-otological imbalance (Fig. 1). Instead, these aetiologies tend to produce lightheadedness or unsteadiness (Table 1, p. 20). Many patients will have evidence of associated cardiovascular and neurological symptoms and signs.

In the absence of auditory symptoms, a thorough history will often uncover a non-otological cause for imbalance. In clinical practice, *cervical spondylosis* and *ageing* are the commonest non-otological causes of unsteadiness. Demyelinating diseases such as multiple sclerosis can also result in disorders of imbalance.

Cervical spondylosis
With increasing age, the cervical spine becomes progressively arthritic, leading to osteophyte formation. These bony growths can constrict the vertebral artery, particularly when the neck is hyperextended, leading to fleeting imbalance due to cerebral ischaemia. It is rare to see any neurological deficits. Management involves a combination of neck physiotherapy and anti-inflammatory drugs.

Ageing
Some degree of imbalance is invariable with the ageing process. The cause is multifactorial, with many of the pathologies shown in Figure 1 presenting simultaneously.

Proprioceptive input is poor due to failing eyesight and hearing. Cervical spondylosis with vertebrobasilar ischaemia is common, and atherosclerosis of cerebral vessels is likely. Additionally, the cardiovascular system may produce postural hypotension and cardiac arrhythmias. Many elderly patients will be on medication that directly or indirectly affects balance, e.g. antihypertensives may cause hypotension.

Vestibular sedatives are best avoided in this group, as they suppress what remains of normal vestibular function, making the problem worse. Attention to eyesight and hearing, the use of a walking stick and a review of drug therapy may lead to symptomatic improvement. Physiotherapy can assist in improved mobility and increased confidence.

Migraine
Although this disease is characterized by a severe hemicranial headache (p. 53), the patient commonly has a feeling of unsteadiness and imbalance. A thorough clinical history will clinch the diagnosis. It is associated with Ménière's disease

Transient ischaemic attacks
A sense of imbalance associated with neurological deficits such as dysarthria, amaurosis fugax and limb weakness can be caused by transient ischaemic attacks. The symptoms are due to microemboli in the cerebral vessels, leading to brain ischaemia. The symptoms and signs resolve within 24 hours, but may herald a cerebrovascular accident.

Head injury (without temporal bone fracture)
Concussion of the central vestibular mechanism can lead to a variety of imbalance symptoms, from initial vertigo to unsteadiness in the recovery phase. Vestibular rehabilitation exercises will improve recovery, although their use may be limited by past injury and neck pain.

Epilepsy
The history should make the diagnosis clear-cut in patients suffering from epilepsy. There is an initial aura followed by loss of consciousness, fitting and, frequently, double incontinence.

Hyperventilation
Unsteadiness attributed to hyperventilation and anxiety is common in young adults. It is often accompanied by tinnitus and tingling in the hands and feet. These patients may require psychological counselling, tranquillizers and, occasionally, beta blockers.

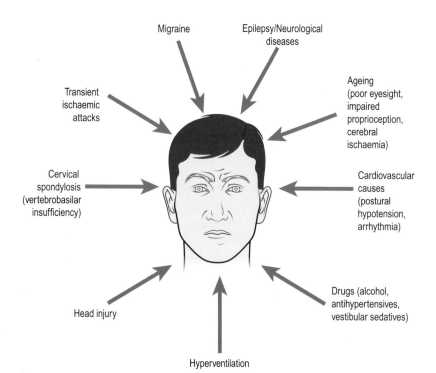

Fig. 1 **Non-otological causes of imbalance are very common.** In the elderly, minor pathological causes can act synergistically to give considerable symptoms.

Disorders of balance – *Non-otological causes*

- Prolonged use of vestibular sedatives may cause imbalance due to labyrinthine suppression
- Imbalance in the elderly is commonly non-otological and multifactorial.

Tinnitus

Noises in the ear, real or imagined, are called tinnitus. This condition affects about 10% of the UK population and is most common in patients who have been exposed to long-term, high-intensity noise. The temporomandibular joint, Eustachian tube and carotid artery can all produce sounds which are usually innocent and classified as objective forms of tinnitus, referred to as somatosounds (Fig. 1).

Aetiology and clinical presentation

Subjective causes of tinnitus (heard only by the patient) are extremely common and the majority of them are treated conservatively (Fig. 1). Otoscopy and audiology will identify the majority of middle ear conditions causing tinnitus (Table 1), which when corrected may improve the symptoms. Very few tinnitus sufferers need detailed investigation. However, unilateral symptoms, particularly if accompanied by hearing loss, should have a full neuro-otological assessment, including an MRI scan.

The commonest form of subjective tinnitus is a rushing, hissing or buzzing noise; it is frequently associated with sensorineural hearing loss. The patient may be unaware of the hearing loss, especially if it is a high-frequency deficit of moderate severity. The character of the tinnitus may give a clue to the aetiology (Table 2).

Presbyacusis (p. 9) is a common cause of tinnitus. Due to the gradual onset, the patient may be unaware of the noise until a heavy cold produces a temporary conductive hearing loss, highlighting the tinnitus.

Certain drugs such as aspirin, alcohol and quinine can exacerbate tinnitus. Ototoxic drug combinations, e.g. aminoglycoside and loop diuretics, can cause permanent symptoms.

Management

Patients with intrusive tinnitus often worry about serious intracranial disease, which serves to reinforce their perception of the noise. It is important therefore that careful explanation and, if necessary, investigation, are undertaken to reassure the sufferer. All hearing deficits should be corrected, either with a hearing aid or (occasionally) surgery. Certain patients find relief by using a tinnitus masking device. This is a noise generator which can be combined with a hearing aid to 'cover up' the patient's tinnitus. While the majority of patients can come to terms with tinnitus, there is a group who require considerable support to overcome their 'disability'. Psychotherapy can help identify stressful factors which exacerbate the symptoms. Counselling and group meetings at a tinnitus association can help to relieve isolation.

Table 1 Ear diseases known to be associated with subjective tinnitus

Location	Disease
External ear	Wax
Middle ear	Otosclerosis
	Middle ear effusion
Inner ear	Noise-induced hearing loss
	Prebycusis
	Menière's disease
	Trauma (surgery, head injury)
	Ototoxic drugs
	Labyrinthitis
	Acoustic neuroma

Table 2 The quality of tinnitus and its likely site of origin

Quality of tinnitus	Site of pathology
High pitched, hissing or rushing	Inner ear, brain stem, auditory cortex
Banging, crackling, popping	Middle ear
Pulsatile	Normal carotid artery, vascular tumour

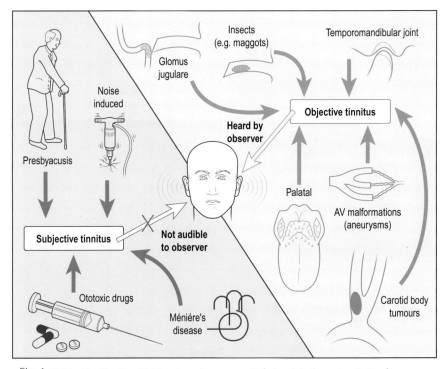

Fig. 1 **Subjective tinnitus.** This is extremely common. Unfortunately, the vast majority of cases are untreatable. **Objective tinnitus.** Most forms of objective tinnitus are readily identifiable and potentially curable. The commonest form is the normal pulsatile noise of blood passing through the internal carotid artery. It is most apparent at night with the ear placed on a pillow.

Tinnitus

- Many tinnitus sufferers are managed by simple reassurance.

- Unilateral tinnitus, particularly if associated with a hearing deficit, should be fully investigated.

- Tinnitus associated with sensorineural hearing loss is best treated with a hearing aid.

- Tinnitus maskers provide effective control for 30% of sufferers.

- Objective causes of tinnitus are rare. The commonest is transmitted noise from the carotid artery.

The auricle (pinna) and ear wax

The auricle (pinna)

Congenital abnormalities

The auricle develops from six separate hillocks on the side of the embryo's head. Minor congenital abnormalities are not uncommon, and most do not require treatment (Fig. 1). Major abnormalities include a complete absence of the pinna (anotia) or severe deformities (Fig. 2). Severe malformations of the pinna and ear canal are not always associated with abnormalities of the middle or inner ear, as these two elements have separate embryological origins. Indeed, many children may have a conductive hearing loss but normal inner ear function.

The results of surgical correction of these auricular defects have been generally unsatisfactory. The recent development of titanium implants, however, allows excellent cosmetic prostheses to be anchored to the mastoid (Fig. 3). As well as providing an anchor, the titanium parts can also act as the transmitter for a bone conduction hearing aid (p. 11).

Bat ears

Bat ears are the commonest abnormalities of the auricle and are usually bilateral (Fig. 4). Prominent ears may be moulded at birth (within 24 hours), as the cartilage has not formed its 'memory' for shape. Surgical correction, however, is best left until about 6–7 years and is designed to recreate an antihelical fold.

Preauricular sinus

The preauricular sinus is an embryological remnant which appears as a small pit anterior to the helical root. No intervention is required unless the sinus becomes infected (Fig. 5). Treatment involves complete excision of the sinus tract to avoid recurrence.

Collaural fistula

A collaural fistula is a rare developmental abnormality in which a tract runs between a pit in the ear canal and the neck skin. It invariably needs excision because of recurrent infection. This may require an extensive dissection of the facial nerve as the tract may pass between nerve branches.

Infections and other conditions

Otitis externa may spread to involve the skin and cartilage of the pinna. Treatment with astringents and

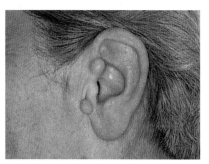

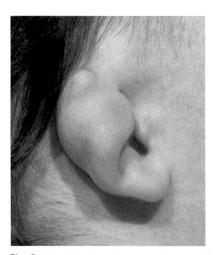

Fig. 1 **Accessory auricles.** These are located along a line from the tragus to the angle of the mouth. They contain cartilage remnants.

Fig. 2 **Microtia of the pinna showing a small severely deformed appendage.**

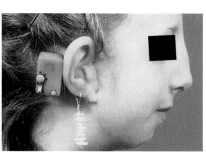

(a)

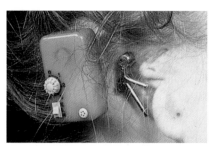

(b)

Fig. 3 **Bone-anchored auricular prosthesis and hearing aid in patient with Treacher Collins syndrome (a).** This is an hereditary condition causing hearing loss, usually due to abnormalities of the external ear including atresia of the ear canal and auricular defects **(b)**. The metal supports for an auricular prosthesis are clearly shown anchored into the skull. Note the excellent cosmetic appearance of the prosthetic auricle.

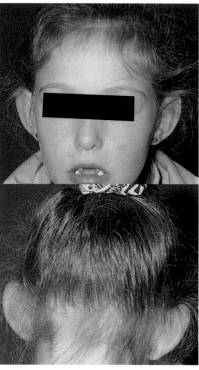

Fig. 4 **Prominent or 'bat' ears.**

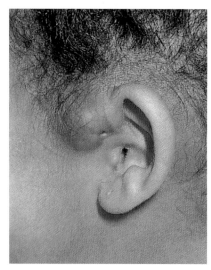

Fig. 5 **An infected preauricular sinus.** The small opening is clearly visible at the root of the helix.

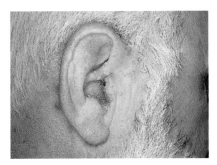

Fig. 6 **Psoriatic eruption affecting both the pinna and the external ear canal.**

systemic antibiotics is needed. Streptococcal infection (erysipelas) is recognized easily by a sharply demarcated 'serpiginous' edge which rapidly spreads. The patient is often toxic, but the response to penicillin is rapid.

Dermatitis from nickel jewellery or eardrops is usually localized to the lobule and concha, respectively. Resolution is rapid if the sensitizing agent is removed. Eczematous and psoriatic eruptions of the auricular skin are not uncommon and will require application of topical creams and ointments (Fig. 6).

Perichondritis is an inflammation of the auricular perichondrium and produces a diffusely swollen, shiny and painful ear. Trauma, otitis externa or surgery may be the cause. Aggressive treatment with broad-spectrum antibiotics, astringents and analgesics is needed to prevent suppuration and cartilage necrosis. This may prevent an ugly, long-term cosmetic defect (cauliflower ear).

Other conditions affecting the auricle include:

■ auricular haematoma (p. 26)
■ tumours (p. 114).

Ear wax

Ear wax contains sebaceous material and the products of the ceruminous glands which line the outer one-third of the ear canal. These secretions combine with desquamated skin and hair to form wax, about which many patients develop an obsession. Wax (cerumen) varies in colour and consistency, and its production appears to be partly controlled by circulating catecholamines. It is normal to have some cerumen in the ear canal. Wax provides protection to the skin and also possesses bactericidal activity. Ear canal epithelium migrates

outwards, providing a natural cleaning mechanism for desquamated tissue and cerumen. Attempts to clean the ear by a patient invariably force the ear canal contents deeper into the meatus (Fig. 7). Wax impaction therefore is a common cause of hearing loss. If water enters the ear, the desquamated keratin expands, often trapping fluid in the deep meatus. This may cause an otitis externa unless the plug is removed.

Removal of wax
Meatal occlusion, impaction, irritation, hearing loss or otitis externa and clinical inspection of the eardrum are all indications for removing wax. The simplest method is to syringe the ear. Tap water at body temperature is used. The pinna is lifted to straighten the ear canal and the water jet aimed at the roof of the canal, never directly at the eardrum. The canal and drum head must be examined afterwards. Patients who have perforations should not have their ears syringed (Table 1). Curetting wax from the canal requires a good light and a cerumen scoop or hoop. In difficult or refractory cases a microscope and sucker may be used in outpatients, or under general anaesthesia. Hard impacted wax may need to be softened with topical ceruminolytic ear drops prior to removal (p. 28).

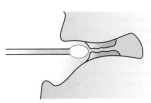

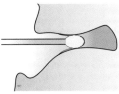

Sound transmission reduced

Fig. 7 **Insertion of cotton buds into the external ear canal to clear wax results in debris being pushed deeper into the meatus.**

Table 1 **Complications of wax removal**

Incomplete removal
Trauma to ear canal skin
Perforation of eardrum
Vertigo (caloric effect in the presence of perforated eardrum or mastoid cavity)

Keratotis obturans
Keratin may desquamate abnormally in the deep meatus to produce a hard ball of debris which is difficult to remove. If left, the ear canal becomes expanded and granulation tissue forms at the margin of the plug. This is a form of cholesteatoma involving the ear canal. Removal is often only possible under a general anaesthetic. Frequent review is necessary to prevent recurrence.

'Attic' wax (attic crust)
Chronic suppurative ottitis media (atticoantral) with cholesteatoma in the attic can appear on inspection to resemble wax above the malleus handle. This is referred to as 'attic' wax (Fig. 8). Removal is usually painful and may induce vertigo. The true nature of the problem is revealed once the cholesteatoma is visualized deep to the wax crust.

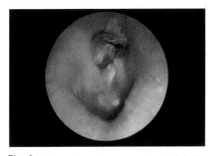

Fig. 8 **Otoscopic appearance of wax debris in the posterior attic (attic crust) which was concealing a cholesteatoma.**

The auricle (pinna) and ear wax

■ Malformations of the pinna and ear canal are not always associated with abnormalities in the middle and inner ear.

■ Perichondritis requires aggressive treatment with broad-spectrum antibiotics, astringents and analgesics to prevent suppuration and cartilage necrosis.

■ Wax in the ear canal is normal.

■ Discourage the use of cotton buds to clear wax debris.

■ Remove soft wax by syringing; hard wax will require prior softening.

■ Do not syringe the ear in the presence of a perforated eardrum.

■ Beware of the 'attic wax crust': it may conceal an underlying cholesteatoma associated with chronic suppurative otitis media.

Otological trauma and foreign bodies

Injuries to the pinna

Auricular haematoma

Blunt trauma to the ear may produce a haematoma. Bleeding occurs deep to the perichondrium, which is stripped from the underlying cartilage so that the ear becomes swollen and the normal architecture of the folds lost (Fig. 1). As the cartilage depends on the perichondrium for survival, necrosis and subsequent scar formation will produce the typical 'cauliflower ear'.

Treatment requires aspiration of the haematoma with a large bore needle under sterile conditions. A firm pressure dressing is applied for 24 hours and the ear re-examined. Re-aspiration may be necessary for some days. Unfortunately, haematomas often clot and cannot be aspirated. In such cases the blood is curetted out after raising a skin flap. Pressure is then applied for several days and antibiotics administered to prevent infection. Aggressive treatment will avoid the late, ugly cosmetic defect.

Lacerations

As the pinna has an excellent blood supply, it is always worth suturing severe lacerations and any avulsed tissue. Exposed cartilage should be trimmed back before closing the skin. Human bites to the pinna tend to become infected. Perichondritis may be prevented by dressing the wound and delaying primary closure for 2–3 days.

The ear lobe may be split by avulsion of an earring in a pierced ear. If sutured directly, these injuries produce an unsightly notched lobe. They should be repaired by a stepped incision with a suture loop to reconstruct the hole.

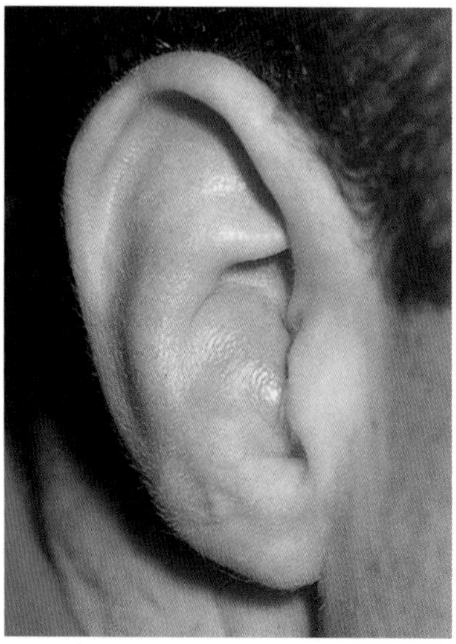

Keloid scars

Keloid scars are common on the ear lobes, particularly in black-skinned people. They can grow to considerable sizes. The aetiology is an exaggerated healing response producing excess collagen outside the original boundaries of the scar. Treatment is difficult. Simple excision usually produces a recurrence. Compression with a silicone gel clip and steroid injections show some success. Large refractory scars may need excision and local radiotherapy.

Injuries to the external meatus

Injuries to the external meatus are almost exclusively due to insertion of foreign bodies into the ear (see opposite). The proverbial matchstick to clear wax is a common culprit. Incorrect insertion of a syringe for dewaxing the ear, or clumsy performance of aural suction are iatrogenic causes. The injury, usually a laceration, is located at the isthmus of the external auditory canal.

Deep injuries can result in perforations of the tympanic membrane and even ossicular chain disruption.

Injuries to the middle and inner ear

The middle and inner ear may both be damaged by either blast injury, barotrauma, head injury or surgical trauma.

Blast injuries

Blast injuries may be produced by either explosions or a simple slap on the ear. There may be multiple sites of damage, depending on the intensity of the pressure wave. The typical injury produces a tympanic membrane rupture. The cochlea may be damaged, resulting in a sensorineural hearing loss and tinnitus, both of which may be permanent. Imbalance occurs if the vestibular apparatus is affected.

Otitic barotrauma

Otitic barotrauma can produce otalgia with some extravasation of blood into the middle ear so that a haemotympanum occurs (Fig. 2). In severe cases the eardrum may rupture. The aetiology is an inability to ventilate the middle ear due to abnormal function of the Eustachian tube. The condition is particularly seen when the ambient pressure is rising, e.g. descent in flight or scuba diving. Treatment comprises a repeated Valsalva manoeuvre to open up the Eustachian tube, in addition to topical nasal decongestants. Myringotomy may be needed in some cases. Patients who fly and suffer regularly are instructed to use prophylactic measures to prevent Eustachian tube problems (e.g. topical nasal decongestants and repeated swallows). Occasionally insertion of a ventilation tube overcomes the problem.

Head injuries

Head injuries may be associated with temporal bone fractures (p. 42). These cause hearing loss, which may be sensorineural if the fracture line passes through the cochlea. In such cases vertigo and facial paralysis may also be present. However, otological trauma can occur in head injuries without the presence of a fracture. The cochlea can be concussed and produce a hearing loss. Labyrinthine damage may lead to benign paroxysmal positional vertigo or a vague feeling of imbalance. Lesions of the central vestibular apparatus can lead to long-term symptoms if compensation is not complete.

Surgical trauma

Surgical trauma may produce a conductive or sensorineural hearing loss. This is a risk in all ear operations, but particularly in stapedectomy where

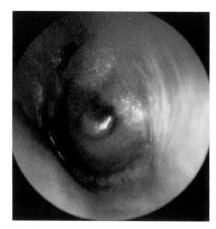

Fig. 1 **An auricular haematoma caused by a rugby football injury.**

Fig. 2 **Blood in the middle ear (haemotympanum).** Causes include otitic barotrauma, secretory otitis media and high jugular bulb.

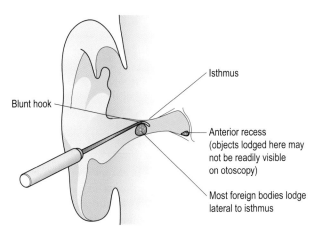

Fig. 3 **Common sites at which foreign bodies become lodged.**

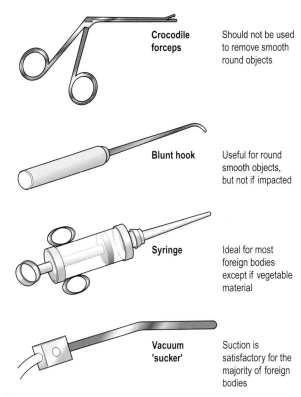

Fig. 4 **Instruments used in the removal of aural foreign bodies.**

the inner ear is deliberately entered, or in mastoid surgery where a cholesteatoma may have disrupted the ossicular chain and invaded the cochlea. The facial nerve is also at risk during middle ear procedures.

Foreign bodies

Children, rather than adults, are most liable to insert foreign bodies into the ear. Not uncommonly they will have also inserted them into the nose. The child usually presents due to parental concern that a foreign body has been lodged in the ear. If insertion passed unnoticed, it may first present with otorrhoea or otalgia. Children generally deny the history. In adults, the usual culprit is an object such as a cotton bud or piece of wood stick employed to dewax the ear.

Most foreign bodies will lodge either lateral to the isthmus (the narrowest part of the ear canal) or impact at that site (Fig. 3). However, if located in the deep meatus they may reside in the anterior recess and therefore not be seen on routine otoscopy. Always check both ears and the nose for foreign bodies in children.

Satisfactory removal of aural foreign bodies requires skill, instruments and optimal lighting. If the clinician does not possess all these then the patient should be referred to a specialist. For most patients, but especially children, repeated attempts at removal are unkind. It is safer to give a general anaesthetic than risk trauma to the external canal or tympanic membrane.

The method of removal depends on the type of foreign body (Figs 4 & 5) and its location. A pair of crocodile forceps can easily grasp objects such as cotton wool, paper and pieces of foam sponge. Forceps should not be employed to grasp smooth round objects as they are likely to spring out of the jaws and end up deeper in the meatus. A blunt hook may be inserted around the object, particularly if round, and gently teased out (Fig. 3). Suction apparatus is also a useful tool in certain cases, e.g. cosmetic beads.

Syringing may be employed in removing non-vegetable foreign bodies. If this method is used for vegetable substances, e.g. rice grains or peas, the object will swell and impact in the ear canal, resulting in severe otalgia.

Occasionally animal foreign bodies such as fleas, ants or flies may enter the external ear canal, causing distressing tinnitus. The creature is killed by instillation of either alcohol or spirit and then may be syringed or suctioned out.

Very rarely the foreign body may be located in the middle ear. This will require a formal opening into the middle ear (tympanotomy) for extraction.

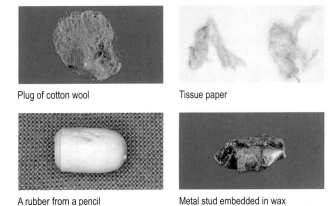

Plug of cotton wool   Tissue paper

A rubber from a pencil   Metal stud embedded in wax

Fig. 5 **A selection of foreign bodies removed from the ear.**

Otological trauma and foreign bodies

- An auricular haematoma or suspected perichondritis requires urgent treatment to avoid a long-term cosmetic defect.

- Head injuries without a fracture can produce severe cochleovestibular symptoms.

- Avoid medical litigation by preoperatively informing patients undergoing ear operations of potential risks to the hearing, balance and facial movement.

- Most foreign bodies lodged in the ear canal are asymptomatic.

- Attempt removal only if you have the skills and instruments.

- It is frequently safer to remove foreign bodies in children under general anaesthesia..

- Do not use forceps to extract smooth round objects.

- Do not syringe out vegetable foreign bodies as they will swell and impact in the ear canal.

Aural drops

There are numerous preparations of aural drops (Table 1).

Table 1 Topical aural preparations
Wax softeners (ceruminolytics)
Olive oil
Sodium bicarbonate
Hydrogen peroxide
Glycerine and urea
Astringents (anti-inflammatory)
Betamethasone
Aluminium acetate
Glycerin and ichthammol
Antibacterial agents
Usually aminoglycosides, combined with anti-Inflammatory agents, e.g.
— Gentisone HC (gentamycin and hydrocortisone)
— Sofradex (framycetin and dexamethasone)
Antifungal agents
Clotrimazole
Econazole
Nystatin

Ceruminolytics

Ceruminolytics, or wax softening agents, are widely used, but many are irritant to the ear canal and should be employed for short periods only. Warm olive oil and bicarbonate are the cheapest solutions. The most expensive preparations contain mixtures, e.g. glycerine, urea and peroxide, but are no more effective than the simple solutions.

Astringents

Astringent aural drops are indicated for otitis externa where the ear canal is oedematous. They assist in reducing the swelling, thereby permitting aural toilet. Subsequent topical antibiotic drops are then more effective. The astringent can be applied on an expanding otowick inserted into the ear canal. Alternatively, the agent may be massaged into a strip of ribbon gauze which is then gently pushed into place.

Antibacterial agents

Antibacterial agents are usually combined with a steroid and should be used for purulent infections. The steroid content is probably the component that is most effective in combating inflamed middle ear mucosa and chronic ear disease. Although most of these drops contain ototoxic agents, many otolaryngologists recommend them for short periods of 7–14 days for discharging grommets or exacerbations of chronic ear disease. However, due to cases of total deafness following such administration, the use of potentially ototoxic agents is *not* recommended in cases where the eardrum is not intact. Prolonged use may cause a secondary fungal growth or contact dermatitis of the ear canal.

Antifungal agents

Otomycosis (usually *Aspergillus* or *Candida* species) invariably results from overuse of antibacterial eardrops and is difficult to treat. The ear canal must be kept meticulously clean and dry. Clotrimazole, econazole and nystatin can be applied topically as drops, cream or powder.

Instillation of aural drops

The maximum benefit of aural drops can only be gained if they are correctly instilled (Fig. 1). If possible, any canal debris should be cleaned prior to their use; this is particularly important in cases of otitis externa.

Instillation of drops is best done by another person. The patient should lie down with the affected ear uppermost. The pinna should be gently lifted upwards and away from the side of the head and the drops introduced. Tragal massage should be used to displace drops as far as the deep meatus and into the middle ear via a perforation or grommet if required. The subject remains in this position for, say, 2–3 minutes. Cotton wool is placed in the ear for half an hour afterwards.

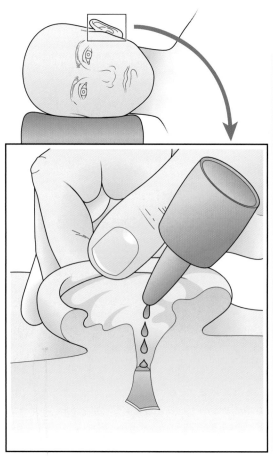

Step 1 Patient lies with ear to be treated uppermost

Step 2 A second person pulls the pinna upwards and outwards

Step 3 The external meatus is filled with aural drops. This invariably means more than five drops, usually 8–10. Mastoid cavities and perforated eardrums may require even more.

Step 4 The tragus should be massaged several times to displace the drops towards the middle ear

Step 5 Remain in position for 2–3 mins

Step 6 Place cotton wool in ear and ask the patient to rise. The cotton wool can be removed 20–30 minutes later

Step 7 Repeat process in other ear if required

Fig. 1 **Topical aural drops are only of any efficacy if instilled correctly as shown above.**

> *Aural drops*
>
> - Simple wax softeners are the most effective, i.e. warm olive oil or sodium bicarbonate.
>
> - Long-term use of topical antibacterial drops can predispose to fungal infection and contact dermatitis.
>
> - Aural drops are only effective if correctly applied. Give the patient precise instructions on the procedure for instillation.

Nose and Paranasal Sinuses

Anatomy and physiology

The nose

In early hominids, the major function of the nose was olfaction, as it still remains in lower mammals. Through the process of evolution, this role has diminished, leading to modification of the internal nasal anatomy of the human nose. Olfaction in modern humans is now sited in a relatively small area high in the nasal vault, and the turbinate structures have become considerably shrunken in size.

Anatomy

It is useful to consider the anatomy of the nose by dividing it into:

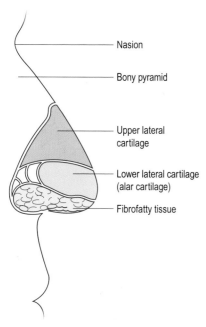

Fig. 1 **Constituent elements of the external nose.**

- the external nose
- the nasal cavity including the nasal septum.

External nose

The upper third of the external nose (Fig. 1) is bony, consisting of nasal bones which connect with the nasion at the forehead. The inferior two-thirds are cartilaginous, consisting of the upper lateral and lower lateral (alar) cartilages. The tip laterally contains resilient but pliable fibrocartilage. This allows maintenance of nasal shape after minor trauma. The skin over the cartilaginous portion is closely adherent and contains multiple sebaceous glands; these latter structures may hypertrophy to form a rhinophyma.

Nasal cavity

The nasal cavity stretches from the vestibule anteriorly to the nasopharynx posteriorly and is divided by a midline osteocartilaginous septum. The lateral wall of the cavity supports a series of ridges called *turbinates* (Fig. 2). These structures are lined by ciliated columnar epithelium and contain erectile tissue. The paranasal sinuses – maxillary, frontal, ethmoid and sphenoid – drain into the nasal cavity around the middle turbinate.

The nasal septum comprises bony and cartilaginous elements. Inferiorly, it is inserted into a groove in the maxillary crest (Fig. 3). It is lined with *mucoperichondrium* and *mucoperiosteum* over the cartilage and bone, respectively. The nasal septum is rarely straight; marked displacement causes nasal airway blockage and an external cosmetic deformity.

Vascular and nerve supply

Both the external and internal carotid arteries supply the nose via their terminal branches. As a guideline, the region above the root of the middle turbinate is supplied by the anterior and posterior ethmoidal arteries, with the remaining areas being supplied by the sphenopalatine, palatine and labial arteries. The carotid system anastomoses at the anteroinferior region of the septum called 'Little's area' or 'Kiesselbach's plexus'.

Venous drainage of the external nose is of importance, as blood can drain via the facial and ophthalmic veins to the cavernous sinus. Therefore, a superficial infection of the nasal lining may involve the carvenous sinus.

The main sensory supply is via the maxillary division of the trigeminal nerve. Secretory glands are under the control of the autonomic nervous system in the vidian nerve. The nasal vascular supply is constricted by sympathetic nerve stimulation and dilated by parasympathetic.

Physiology

Filtration and protection

Particulate matter in inspired air is initially trapped by the *vibrissae* in the nasal vestibule. For any smaller size material, e.g. pollen, the *mucus blanket* provides a tacky surface to which

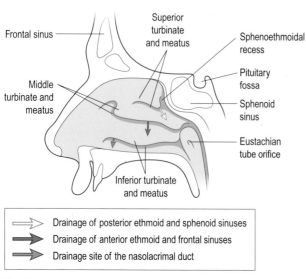

Drainage of posterior ethmoid and sphenoid sinuses
Drainage of anterior ethmoid and frontal sinuses
Drainage site of the nasolacrimal duct

Fig. 2 **Structure of the lateral wall of the nasal cavity.**

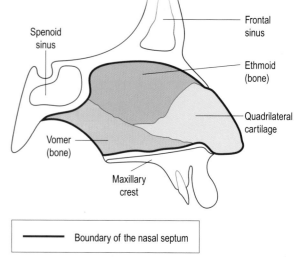

Boundary of the nasal septum

Fig. 3 **The nasal septum.**

adherence occurs. This is transported posteriorly by the beating action of the *nasal cilia*, at a rate of 5–6 mm/min. A volume of 300–500 mL is swallowed daily. A defect in this ciliary action is the cardinal feature of the rare Kartagener's syndrome, in which patients present with rhinorrhoea, chronic secretory otitis media, chronic sinusitis, bronchiectasis and dextrocardia.

Glycoproteins, enzymes such as lysozyme, together with IgA and IgG provide additional passive protection.

Humidification and warming
Excessive drying and extremes of temperature will prevent normal ciliary action. Normally, the inspired air is heated to about 30°C and to about 95% relative humidity. Any variation may severely affect the functioning of the nose and the lower respiratory tract. The profuse vascular supply and numerous secretory glands provide the nose with the necessary structures to prevent any gross variation of these optimal parameters.

Olfaction
Since the specialized olfactory mucosa is located high in the nasal vault, a sniff is required to enhance the appreciation of odours. Additionally, the air must be moist. Physical obstruction, such as a deviated septum or inflammatory swelling, will prevent air reaching the desired site. Viral infections may damage the delicate olfactory nerve endings, and severe trauma can transect the nerve fibres as they traverse the cribriform plate. As with all special senses, acuity diminishes with age.

Vocal resonance
The individual quality of the voice is imparted by the size and form of the nasal cavity. Vocal quality is impaired if the nose becomes blocked, and this may be a serious handicap to professional voice users, particularly singers. Clearly, nasal operations have the potential to also alter vocal resonance and hence voice quality.

The paranasal sinuses

Anatomy
The paranasal sinuses (Fig. 4) are really extensions of the nasal cavity as air-filled spaces into the skull bones. Although paired anatomically, from a pathophysiological view they should be grouped as anterior and posterior. The frontal, anterior ethmoidal and maxillary sinuses (anterior group) drain into the *middle meatus*, and the posterior ethmoidal and sphenoid (posterior group) drain into the *superior meatus* and *sphenoethmoidal recess*. The crucial drainage area of the anterior group of paranasal sinuses is called the *ostiomeatal complex* (Fig. 4). The nasolacrimal duct opens into the anterior part of the inferior meatus.

Frontal sinus
The frontal sinus is not present at birth, but when fully developed may be extensively pneumatized. Its important boundaries are the orbit and anterior cranial fossa. It drains via the region of the ethmoidal–ostiomeatal complex, before entering the nasal cavity.

Maxillary sinus
Although present at birth, the maxillary sinus continues to grow until the early part of the third decade. Anatomical landmarks to be noted include the close relationship of the orbit, teeth, nasal cavity and cheek. These sites can be affected by pathology in the maxillary sinus, and vice versa.

Ethmoid sinus
The ethmoid sinuses describe a labyrinth of air-filled cavities located in the superior and lateral part of the nose rather like a honeycomb. The walls are very thin, thus allowing easy spread of infection and tumour to adjacent structures such as the orbit through the lamina papyracea, and the anterior cranial fossa via the cribriform plate.

Sphenoid sinus
Rapid development of the sphenoid sinus occurs at puberty. The main significance of this sinus is the important structures adjacent, including the internal carotid artery, optic nerve and cavernous sinus. The last contains the oculomotor, trochlear and abducent nerves, as well as the 1st and 2nd divisions of the trigeminal. The pituitary fossa lies posteriorly. The sphenoid sinus is divided by a septum.

Physiology
No specific function has been attributed to the paranasal sinuses. The following have been considered:

- an aid to vocal resonance
- reduction of skull weight
- protection of the eye from trauma
- protection of vital intracranial structures.

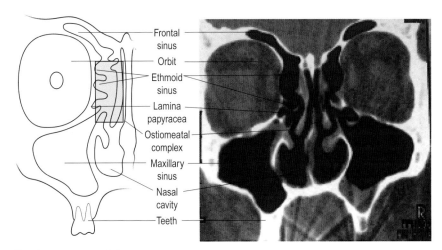

Fig. 4 **The paranasal sinuses.**

Anatomy and physiology

- The nose is structurally composed of bone and cartilage.
- Both the external and internal carotid arteries provide the rich vascular supply of the nasal mucosa.
- The nose has an important protective role in filtering, humidifying and warming inspired air.
- The nose, as part of the respiratory tract, is prone to acute infection and allergic phenomena.
- Since the paranasal sinuses drain via the nose, sinus disease is frequently due to primary problems in the nose.

Symptoms, signs and investigations

Symptoms

It is vital to establish the *precise* complaint of the patient; thus, a full history is mandatory (Fig. 1).

Nasal obstruction

Nasal obstruction is probably the most common symptom, and may be due to anatomical abnormalities, disorders of the mucous membrane lining or stimulation of the autonomic nervous system (Table 1). An allergic aetiology is frequently volunteered by the patient where the symptoms manifest after contract with allergens such as grass pollen, feathers or animal furs. Viral infections, e.g. acute coryza and influenza, cause severe nasal obstruction but generally resolve rapidly over days. An overactivity of the parasympathetic as compared to the sympathetic nerve supply will cause dilatation of the vascular tree and hence engorgement. This is particularly noted by some patients in stress situations and with alterations in ambient temperature and humidity. Neoplasia produces a progressive obstruction and may cause ocular and dental problems due to contiguous spread.

Nasal discharge

The specific character of a nasal discharge is very helpful in deciding aetiology (Table 2). Many patients describe this symptom as 'catarrh'. However, if it produces a runny nose, the discharge should be described as rhinorrhoea and the term 'catarrh' (or postnasal drip) reserved for complaints of nasal discharge passing backwards into the nasopharynx. *Epistaxis* is defined as nasal haemorrhage and is most commonly due to spontaneous

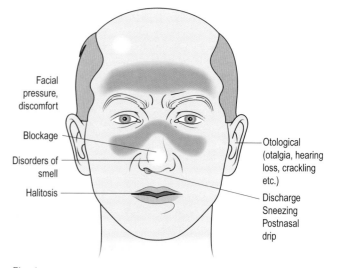

Fig. 1 **Symptoms in nasal and paranasal sinus disease.**

rupture of a blood vessel in the nasal mucous membrane. However, it is vital to exclude any bleeding disorders and neoplasms. If the discharge is offensive, it may indicate a bacterial infection, the presence of a foreign body or neoplasia.

Sneezing

Sneezing is a very frequent accompaniment of allergic and infective rhinitis. Commonly, patients with allergies to household dust and dust mite sneeze on awakening, as the bed mattress forms a huge reservoir of these allergens.

Facial pressure/pain

It is relatively uncommon to see facial pain due to a local cause such as nasal vestibulitis or herpes eruption. More frequently it is related to disease in the distribution of the trigeminal nerve, which supplies the sensory component to the face and the interior of the nose and paranasal sinus via the ophthalmic and maxillary nerves. Consequently, these anatomical sites require detailed examination in such cases (p. 53).

Otological

Any pathological process that disrupts the proper functioning of the Eustachian tube may give rise to aural symptoms. Nasal polyps, particularly of the antrochoanal variety, can physically block the pharyngeal end of the tube. Allergic diseases result in a similar problem by provoking oedema, and neoplasms may directly invade the Eustachian tube. The most frequent otological symptom is hearing loss

caused by a middle ear effusion secondary to Eustachian tube dysfunction.

Disorders of smell

Anosmia, a total loss of sense of smell, is rare. *Hyposmia*, a reduced sense of smell, is more common.

Cacosmia, which is an unpleasant smell detected mainly by others, may be caused by chronic nasal sepsis. *Ozaena*, a foul smell, is a common complaint in anaerobic infections seen in cases of atrophic rhinitis, but the presence of a foreign body and tumour must be excluded.

Halitosis

Poor dental hygiene and poor diet are the most common causes of halitosis. However, chronic sinusitis with purulent postnasal drip can also produce this symptom (p. 51).

Signs

A comprehensive approach to examination of the nose can only be acquired by practice. It is essential to examine both the exterior and interior of the nose, and also ancillary areas such as the ears and oropharynx.

External

Certain cosmetic deformities such as angulation of the bony nasal pyramid or a nasal hump may be obvious. A saddle deformity due to previous injury or infection is readily identified, and it is not unusual to find the septal

---

Table 1 **Causes of nasal obstruction**

Variety	Associated conditions
Anatomical	Septal deflection
	Adenoidal hypertrophy
	Neoplasia
	Choanal atresia
Disorders of nasal lining	Allergic and infective rhinitis
	Nasal polyps
Autonomic nervous system	Vasomotor rhinitis

Table 2 **Nasal discharge: its characteristics and significance**

Character of discharge	Associated conditions
Watery/mucoid	Allergic, infective (viral) and vasomotor rhinitis
	Cerebrospinal fluid leak
Mucopurulent	Infective (bacterial) rhinitis and sinusitis
	Foreign body
Serosanguineous	Neoplasia
Bloody	Trauma, neoplasia, bleeding diathesis

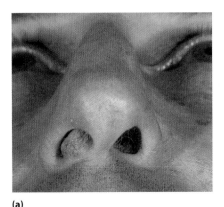

(a)

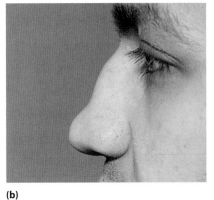

(b)

Fig. 2 **Functional and cosmetic deformities of the nose. (a)** The caudal end of the nasal septum is dislocated into the right nostril. **(b)** Saddle deformity caused by excessive removal of septal cartilage.

cartilage dislocated into the nasal vestibule (Fig. 2).

Internal

A systematic examination is essential to adequately visualize all areas. The inferior turbinate is very prominent and often mistaken for a polyp. Common nasal polyps are white/grey in colour and painless on palpation.

Mucopus in the middle meatus may indicate infection in the anterior group of sinuses.

The postnasal space or nasopharynx is a difficult region to view with a head light and mirror. However, modern flexible instruments and rigid endoscopes have eased the difficulties. The sites to visualize include the Eustachian tube cushions, the posterior choanae, the roof of the nasopharynx, and the fossa of Rosenmüller which is a recess situated immediately posterior to the Eustachian tube.

Examination of the paranasal sinuses is limited to palpation. In an acute frontal sinusitis, there is localized tenderness in the floor of the sinus. Maxillary tumours may cause expansion of the malar and deformities of the teeth-bearing alveolus.

Investigations

Clinical investigations should not replace mandatory history taking and physical examination. Many of the investigations are performed mainly to confirm the diagnosis and rarely add much more information. Nevertheless, critical use and appraisal affords a useful adjunct to history and examination.

Allergy testing

The simplest variety of allergy test is a skin-prick performed on the volar aspect of the forearm. A wide variety of allergens are possible, but the common ones include pollens, animal dander, household dust and dust mite. Controls such as saline and histamine should be employed. A positive response produces a wheal and flare (in about 20 minutes) which can be graded. However, a negative response does not exclude allergy, and a positive response is not absolute proof that the specific allergen is causing symptoms (Fig. 3). The radioallergosorbent test (RAST) measures allergen-specific serum immunoglobulin E, but this technique is expensive and reserved for special cases.

Radiology

Plain views of the sinuses have limited value. CT scanning is the imaging of choice for the majority of nasal and sinus disease (Fig. 4). Soft tissue

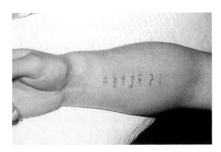

Fig. 3 **A skin-prick test illustrating multiple allergies.**

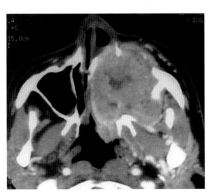

Fig. 4 **CT scan showing a malignant tumour of the maxillary sinus with bone erosion in the nasal cavity and cheek.**

abnormalities and tumours usually require magnetic resonance imaging (MRI) (Fig. 5). MRI distinguishes retained secretions from soft tissue masses.

Mucociliary clearance

Mucociliary clearance can be assessed in cases of suspected ciliary motility disorder, e.g. Kartagener's syndrome. A pellet of saccharin placed on the anterior end of the inferior turbinate should be tasted by the patient in about 20 minutes. Prolongation of this time occurs in some normals after nasal infections and in primary ciliary dyskinesia.

Miscellaneous

Rhinomanometry, which measures nasal air flow and resistance, is a highly specialized research tool. Nasal provocation tests are more accurate than skin tests, but are time consuming as only a single allergen can be tested at a time. Eosinophilia in nasal smears and blood is supportive of a diagnosis of allergic rhinitis.

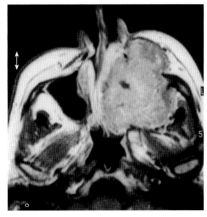

Fig. 5 **MRI scan (T1) complementary to Figure 4: soft tissue detail is enhanced.**

> ### Symptoms, signs and investigations
>
> - Nasal obstruction is the commonest symptom.
> - The characteristics of nasal discharge may be suggestive of particular disease.
> - Nasal pathology may, via the trigeminal nerve, give rise to referred head and neck pain.
> - The internal nose is best examined using a rigid endoscope.
> - Skin-prick tests for nasal allergy are recommended for investigating rhinitis.
> - CT and MRI have replaced plain radiology in the detailed examination of the nose and paranasal sinuses.

Allergic and vasomotor rhinitis

The term 'rhinitis' implies an inflammatory response of the lining membrane of the nose and may be intermittent or persistent. It is important to understand that such an event can occur as a consequence of both primary allergic and non-allergic mechanisms (Fig. 1). In allergic rhinitis, specific allergens are responsible for a type 1 hypersensitivity reaction, and the symptom complex may be subclassified as being predominantly seasonal or perennial. Non-allergic pathologies include viral and bacterial infections (pp. 38, 50), as well as autonomic nervous system abnormalities which can result in vasomotor rhinitis.

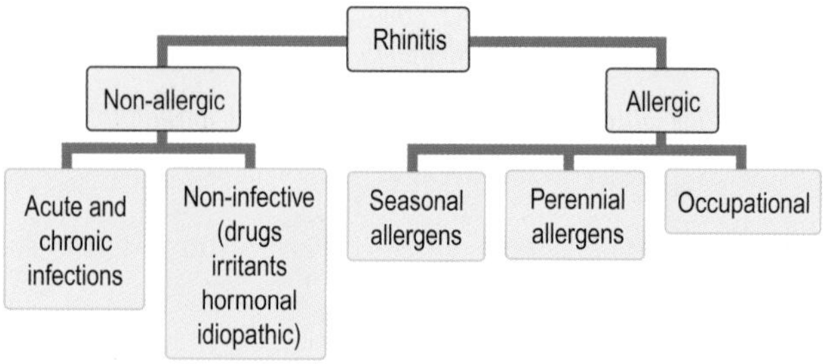

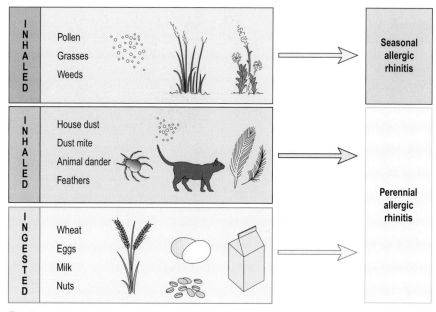

Fig. 1 **Causes of rhinitis.**

Allergic rhinitis

Between 10 and 20% of the population suffer to some degree from nasal manifestations of an antigen–antibody type 1 hypersensitivity reaction (Fig. 2). In seasonal allergic rhinitis (hay fever), the allergens are inhaled, e.g. grass, pollens, weeds and flowers. Animal dander, household dust, the dust mite and feathers are the principal allergens in perennial allergic rhinitis and have no seasonal variation. Rarely, ingested allergens are implicated in the perennial group, e.g. dairy products and wheat.

Clinical features

The clinical features of allergic rhinitis include the classic triad of:

- nasal obstruction due to mucosal vasolidation and oedema
- rhinorrhoea (runny nose) due to enhanced activity of glandular elements
- paroxysms of sneezing due to mucosal stimulation.

The symptom complex is produced by allergen binding to immunoglobulin E (IgE), which in turn is bound to mast cells. This causes degranulation of mast cells and the release of mediator substances such as histamine, leukotrienes and SRSA.

Many patients have associated evidence of atopy such as asthma, eczema, allergic dermatitis and drug allergies. Aspirin sensitivity is not infrequent. Taking a detailed clinical history may identify the allergens involved.

Typically, the nasal mucosa has a boggy, oedematous appearance (Fig. 3); it is covered by a thin layer of watery secretion. Application of a vasoconstrictor produces marked mucosal shrinking with improvement in the nasal airway. Skin-prick tests

Fig. 2 **Common allergens in allergic rhinitis.**

should be interpreted only in relation to the history. Negative skin tests in the face of obvious allergens are not infrequent.

Management

The simplest treatment is avoidance of known allergens. In perennial allergic rhinitis, the quantity of dust and dust mite may be reduced in the bedclothes by:

- changing a feather pillow to foam
- washing the bedclothes twice weekly, as the antigen is heat sensitive

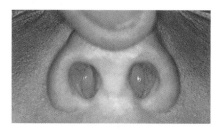

Fig. 3 **Oedematous inferior turbinates narrowing the nasal airway in a patient with hay fever.**

- using commercial sprays that inhibit house dust mite
- using a dust proof cover over the mattress, duvet and pillows
- avoiding carpets and heavy drapes in the bedroom.

Suspected food allergens may be excluded from the diet or replaced with suitable alternatives. Removing animal dander by giving up a pet may be emotionally upsetting but necessary.

Desensitization injections may be offered. These work on the principle of producing a blocking IgG antibody that prevents antigen binding to IgE. Obviously, the treatment is only of value if specific allergens can be identified, and it is essential to commence the series of necessary injections well in advance of the exposure. Due to the risk of anaphylaxis, desensitization must be done in a controlled environment with adequate resuscitation available.

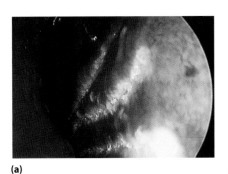

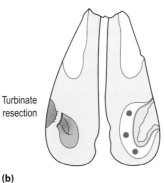

Turbinate resection

● Sites of submucosal diathermy

— Shrunken position of turbinate

(a)   **(b)**

Fig. 4 **(a) Endoscopic photograph of turbinate after laser reduction. (b) Resection and submucosal diathermy of inferior turbinates to relieve obstruction.**

Drug therapy

Therapy involving the use of both topical and systemic drugs has been directed at either preventing mast cell degranulation or blocking the effect of released mediators.

Topical sodium cromoglycate stabilizes the mast cell membrane and prevents the release of chemical agents. It has provided effective relief of asthmatic symptoms but has been less successful in allergic rhinitis. Local decongestants can be either sympathomimetic agents or steroids. The former group includes ephedrine nose drops which provide dramatic shrinkage of nasal mucosa, but long-term use can lead to rhinitis medicamentosa. Locally-acting steroid nasal sprays, e.g. beclometasone, fluticasone, are highly effective against blockage and rhinorrhoea. Regular use in a 'course' is important. Topical antihistamines are an alternative.

Systemic drug therapy includes antihistamines which act by blocking the H_1 nasal mucosa receptors. Their major drawback is drowsiness. Modern derivatives are less able to cross the blood–brain barrier, hence reducing side-effects. If sedation occurs, medication can be taken at night.

Surgery

Surigical treatment (Fig. 4) is only infrequently indicated, as most patients' symptoms are controlled by conservative therapy. Turbinate resection, cautery or outfracture may improve nasal obstruction, but rhinorrhoea and sneezing are unaffected by surgical manipulations.

Intrinsic rhinitis (vasomotor rhinitis)

Intrinsic rhinitis is common (10–15% of the population). The symptoms are similar to allergic rhinitis with less sneezing, and the patient does not have positive allergy testing results. The pathophysiology involves an imbalance between the parasympathetic and sympathetic autonomic nerve supply of the nasal mucosa. The former predominates causing nasal obstruction due to increased vascularity. Enhanced mucosal secretion produces watery rhinorrhoea.

Patients may relate an attack of symptoms to changes in ambient humidity and temperature. Metabolic changes seen in pregnancy, puberty, the menopause and hyperthyroidism can cause the same nasal response. Certain drugs have also been implicated, particularly antihypertensives and the contraceptive pill.

Clinical features

The main clinical features include nasal obstruction, rhinorrhoea and sneezing as in allergic rhinitis. The nasal mucosa over the inferior turbinate is congested, swollen and red, occasionally completely blocking the airway. Some patients may complain that symptoms occur on exposure to sunlight, gaseous irritants such as tobacco or with ingestion of alcohol.

Management

In all but the mildest of cases, medical treatment in the form of local and systemic decongestants should be tried. Severe cases may require submucosal diathermy, laser treatment or radical turbinectomy to clear the nasal airway (Fig. 4).

Rhinitis Medicamentosa

Rhinitis medicamentosa is characterized by reactive vasodilatation of the nasal mucosa. It is a result of acquired sensitivity of the nasal lining to prolonged use of topical agents, particularly those containing sympathomimetic agents. Many 'over the counter' medicines fall into this category. The patient rapidly becomes addicted to the short periods of relief produced from the severe chronic nasal obstruction.

Management

Treatment should be prophylactic, i.e. certain preparations should only be employed as 'short sharp' therapies. Established rhinitis medicamentosa requires substitution of the offending drug by one containing a steroid, or by employing a systemic decongestant. In severe cases, the mucosal swelling becomes irreversible. Such cases require surgical treatment, usually turbinate resection (Fig. 4).

Allergic and vasomotor rhinitis

- The commonest perennial allergens are household dust and dust mite.
- Pollen is the commonest seasonal allergen.
- False-negative results on skin tests are not infrequent.
- Sinofacial congestion is common in allergic rhinitis.
- Rhinitis and asthma frequently coexist as part of the same disease process.
- The mainstay of treatment of allergic and vasomotor rhinitis is medical.
- Topical nasal steroid preparations are valuable in reducing or abolishing the allergic reactions in many patients and can be prescribed long term.
- Prolonged application of potent topical vasoconstrictors leads to rhinitis medicamentosa.

Nasal polyps and foreign bodies

Nasal polyps

The majority of nasal polyps are associated with intrinsic rhinitis and allergy (Table 1), although only about 25% of patients have positive skin-prick tests.

Nasal polyps are 'bags' of oedematous mucosa and most frequently arise from the ethmoid cells and prolapse into the nose via the middle meatus. They are nearly always bilateral. If allowed to grow they may present in the nasal vestibule (Fig. 1). The cardinal symptom is progressive nasal obstruction. Rhinorrhoea is frequent and ocassionally a history of recurrent sinusitis due to ostial blockage is a feature. Otological symptoms and hyposmia may occur.

Chronic sinus infection can result in polypoid mucosal disease which, clinically, produces similar features to idiopathic nasal polyposis.

Clinical features

Examination reveals single or multiple pale, grey polypoid masses which are insensitive to palpation and do not bleed. Unilaterality and haemorrhage should arouse the suspicion of neoplasia. CT scans may reveal radio-opacity due to secondary infection, in the paranasal sinuses, particularly of the maxillary antrum.

Management

Large polys are treated by pernasal removal. Small polyps can be managed by topical nasal steroids. Short-term systemic steroids are also occasionally administered. Recurrence rates may be reduced by long-term topical steroids, post-surgery. Any chronic sinus infection should be treated in conjunction with nasal polypectomy. Rarely, an ethmoidectomy may be

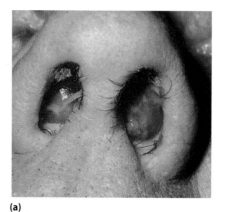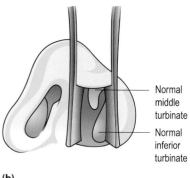

(a) **(b)**

Fig. 1 **Bilateral nasal polyps presenting in the nasal vestibules (a).** A polyp can easily be confused with a normal inferior turbinate **(b)** especially if the turbinate is hypertrophic.

Normal middle turbinate

Normal inferior turbinate

required for frequent recurrences. Routine management strategies for the underlying allergy or asthma should also be instituted (pp. 34–35).

Antrochoanal polyp

The antrochoanal polyp is uncommon. It is usually unilateral and commences as oedematous lining in the maxillary sinus. This prolapses, usually via a posterior accessory ostium, into the nasal cavity and enlarges toward the posterior choana and naspoharynx. The patient, commonly a young adult, complains of unilateral nasal obstruction, which is worse on expiration due to the ball valve effect of the polyp in the posterior choana. If significantly large it may block both choanae and cause otological symptoms due to obstruction of the Eustachian tube (Fig. 2). Patients occasionally present so late that the polyp has

enlarged behind the soft palate and hangs visibly in the oropharynx.

Treatment is surgical by pernasal excision with removal of the cystic antral portion endoscopically via an antrostomy. Recurrences may require a Caldwell–Luc approach to the antrum to remove the roots of the cyst.

Neoplastic polyps

Neoplastic polyps (p. 110) are invariably unilateral and cause progressive symptoms: nasal obstruction, epiphora (blocking of the vasolacrimal duct), epistaxis and foul smelling nasal discharge. They are frequently fleshy in appearance and bleed on palpation. Biopsy is mandatory.

Miscellaneous polyps

Nasal polyps are extremely rare in children. In this age group, careful consideration should be given to any evidence of cystic fibrosis, and a sweat test should be performed.

Prolapse of the meninges (meningocele) or cerebrum (encephalocele) can occur through an anterior cranial fossa defect. This should be excluded radiologically prior to excision or biopsy.

Nasal foreign bodies

Young children (and on occasion, psychiatric cases) are the main patients who insert foreign bodies into the nose. The variety of foreign bodies is protean (Fig. 3), but readily available items such as foam rubber, peas and small stones are frequent. Inorganic objects may be in situ for long periods

Table 1 **Causes of nasal polyps**
Infection
Rhinitis
Sinusitis — chronic paranasal infection
Nasal allergy, e.g. aspirin sensitivity, seasonal and perennial allergic rhinitis
Idiopathic
Neoplasia
Association with other diseases
Asthma
Cystic fibrosis
Bronchiectasis

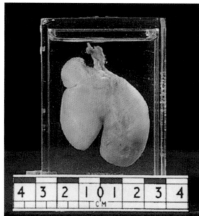

Fig. 2 **Antrochoanal polyp.** A surgical specimen showing the classic dumbbell appearance. This caused total unilateral nasal blockage.

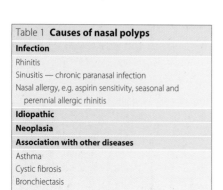

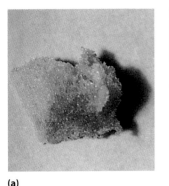
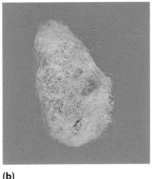
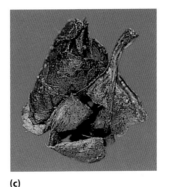
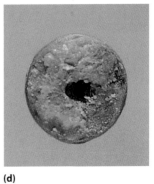

(a) (b) (c) (d)

Fig. 3 **A selection of removed nasal foreign bodies.** (a) Piece of sofa sponge. (b) Piece of cotton wool. (c) Leaf. (d) Rubber pencil end.

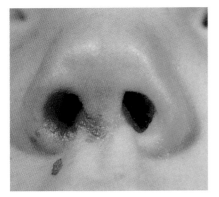

Fig. 4 **Unilateral nasal vestibulitis caused by a nasal foreign body.** The patient presented with a 3-week history of foul odour.

before producing symptoms. However, organic objects, such as paper, wool and vegetable material, produce a brisk mucosal reaction and hence rapid onset of symptoms (Fig. 4).

Clinical features
The child is usually calm, although prior clumsy attempts at removal may have caused distress. Usually, the parents provide a sound history which an older child frequently denies. The cardinal sign is a unilateral nasal discharge which is foul smelling if the foreign body has been present for any length of time (Fig. 4). Excoriation of the nasal vestibular skin and upper lip may be present. The foreign body frequently impacts in the lower part of the nose and on ocassions simply rests in the nasal vestibule. Unless there is a marked infection, visualization is usually possible in good light by elevating the nasal tip gently with the thumb.

Management
In a cooperative child, the foreign body may be either grasped by cupped forceps or flicked out with a blunt hooked probe. An adult may need to restrain a young child. The limbs are usually wrapped in a blanket and the head held steady (Fig. 5). A general

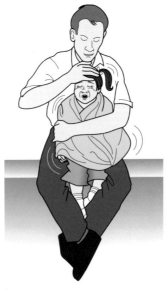

Fig. 5 **Restraining a young child when removing a nasal foreign body.**

anaesthetic will be required in all other instances, as inept attempts could push the object further back with the subsequent risk of inhalation or traumatic haemorrhage. In some instances it is safer to deliver the object via the nasopharynx. The other nostril must be examined to exclude a second foreign body.

Rhinolith
Rhinolith is the term applied to a large foreign body found in the nose of some adults. It is composed of deposits of calcium and magnesium on a nidus such as a piece of gauze or clotted blood. There is frequently a history of nasal packing for epistaxis many years previous (Fig. 6).

Clinical features and management
Nasal obstruction and discharge are the most common symptoms. The latter may be foul smelling and blood-stained due to the presence of infection and friable granulations. Examination reveals a mass that is hard to palpation. Plain radiology can confirm the diagnosis.

Rhinoliths should preferably be removed in one piece, but their sheer bulk may require piecemeal extraction.

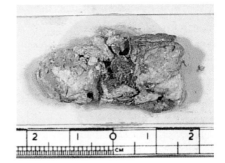

Fig. 6 **Rhinolith.** A large specimen extracted from a patient who had required nasal packing for epistaxis many years previous. The nidus (coloured red) was a remnant of the gauze employed.

Nasal polyps and foreign bodies

- The majority of nasal polyps are usually bilateral, secondary to rhinitis, and painless.
- The prevalence of polyps increases with age.
- Beware of unilateral bleeding polyps. They may be neoplastic and should be biopsied.
- Nasal polyps are extremely rare in children.
- A foul smelling unlateral nasal discharge in a child requires exclusion of a nasal foreign body.
- Beware: foreign bodies can be inhaled.
- Resort to removal under general anaesthesia if the patient is uncooperative, or removal is difficult. The patient will thank you.

Nasal infections

Common cold

In the common cold (acute coryza or acute rhinitis), the nasal mucosa is infected by a virus. Those particularly implicated include:

- adeno- and rhinoviruses
- respiratory syncytial influenzae
- parainfluenzae.

Infection rates appear to be related to an immaturity of the immune system, thereby explaining the increased incidence in children. On average, children suffer from 6–12 infections per year. This may be compounded by other factors which compromise the immune mechanism, such as malnutrition, AIDS and immunosuppressive drugs.

Clinical features

The nasal lining is hyperaemic and the glandular component fiercely stimulated. These changes produce the cardinal symptoms of:

- nasal obstruction
- sneezing
- rhinorrhoea.

Secondary bacterial infections with *Haemophilus influenzae*, streptococcus or staphylococcus species cause mucopurulent nasal discharge. Pyrexia and headache are frequent accompaniments.

Management

The patient should preferably be isolated, as the infection is highly contagious. Treatment is symptomatic as the disease is self-limiting. Steam inhalations and topical nasal decongestants may provide some relief from nasal obstruction. The constitutional symptoms of pyrexia and muscular pains are best controlled by an antipyretic such as a non-steroidal anti-inflammatory or paracetamol. Antibiotics may be required if bacterial complications ensue (Table 1).

Table 1 **Complications of acute coryza**
Secretory otitis media
Acute otitis media
Nasopharyngitis
Acute sinusitis
Cervical lymphadenitis
Laryngitis
Pneumonia

If the secretory glands do not revert to normal, then the patient may be left with a complaint of 'postnasal drip' due to continued mucoid secretion.

Nasal vestibulitis

Excoriation of the skin of the nasal vestibule may be due to a vast array of local and general conditions. In the former category, nose picking, a dislocated columella and rhinorrhoea from nasal allergy are common (Fig. 1). Herpes simplex and zoster vesicles may occur in the anterior nares (Fig. 2). In children, the purulent nasal discharge from a foreign body frequently causes a vestibulitis (Fig. 4, p. 37). Generalized eczema can also affect the nasal vestibule. The commonest bacteria causing vestibulitis are the staphylococci, a commensal in the anterior nares of some individuals (p. 39).

Treatment consists of topical antibiotics and, occasionally, systemic as well, but only after swab cultures have been taken. In eczematous cases,

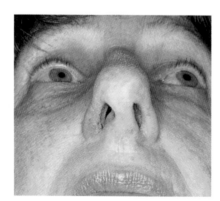

Fig. 1 **Constant rhinorrhoea due to vasomotor rhinitis has resulted in severe vestibulitis compounded by the need to wipe the nose.**

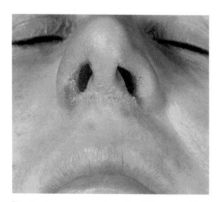

Fig. 2 **A severe nasal vestibulitis caused by herpes simplex infection.**

application of a steroid base ointment may be required.

Persistent vestibulitis with evidence of ulceration may be associated with a neoplastic process such as basal or squamous cell carcinoma.

Atrophic rhinitis

Atrophic rhinitis is characterized by severe crusting in the nasal cavities and atrophy of the surface mucosa and the bony turbinates. If associated with foetor, the term 'ozaena' is employed. Unfortunately, patients are unaware of this foul odour as the pathophysiology renders them anosmic. The precise aetiology is uncertain, but *Pseudomonas* has been implicated. Capacious nasal cavities as a result of nasal surgery may also be a cause. In most cases, poor hygiene and malnutrition are features. Females are most frequently affected. It is very rare in the UK.

Clinical features

The foul stench renders the unfortunate patient socially unacceptable. Vast volumes of crusts are present in the nasal cavities, removal of which causes epistaxis. In extreme cases the crusts fill the nasopharynx and may coat the posterior pharyngeal wall.

Management

Management calls for meticulous local toilet. This is best effected by douching the nose three to four times daily, either with a Higginson syringe or a modern water toothpick (Fig. 3). With the latter, the force of the saline jet can be controlled. Prolonged courses of ciprofloxacin antibiotic are helpful if *Pseudomonas* is cultured.

Surgical techniques are designed to narrow the nasal cavities by interposition of bone or cartilage. If all else fails, the nostril can be surgically closed and reopened months later.

The principle of all treatment policies is to allow an opportunity for the atrophic tissue to regenerate normal ciliated columnar epithelium.

Nasal furunculosis

The organism *Staphylococcus aureus* is the major cause of hair follicle infection in the nasal vestibule, resulting in nasal furunculosis. Some

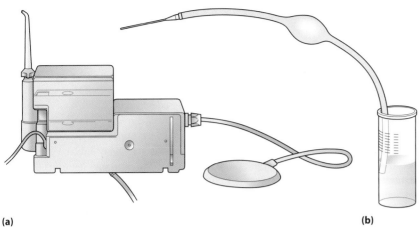

(a) **(b)**

Fig. 3 **Nasal toilet to clear the crusts in atrophic rhinitis may be performed with (a) a modern water toothpick or (b) a traditional 'Higginson syringe'.**

individuals are chronic asymptomatic nasal carriers of this bacterium. Nose picking is a frequent initiator.

The nose is tender to touch and red (Fig. 4). A swab should be taken and the patient commenced on systemic and topical antibiotics. Patients should be advised not to squeeze out pus as there is a potential risk of spreading infection to the cavernous sinus via the facial veins.

Diabetes mellitus should be excluded in cases of recurrent nasal furunculosis.

Specific nasal dermatitides
Specific dermatitides are rare in the nasal vestibule. Occasionally the

condition may be part and parcel of a generalized skin condition, such as psoriasis, seborrhoeic dermatitis and rosacea (Figs 5 & 6). These conditions usually resolve by ensuring the area is kept clean and covered with a steroid antibiotic ointment or barrier cream.

Lupus vulgaris
Lupus vulgaris is an infection with *Mycobacterium tuberculosis* and presents classically as an indolent ulcer of the nasal vestibule and septum.

Lupus pernio
The skin may be involved in sarcoidosis (Boeck's disease). This may manifest as erythema nodosum, which

can be associated with disease of the nasal skin (lupus pernio). In the nose these present as bluish-red nodules (Fig. 7).

Sarcoidosis is a systemic disease so that other tissues are invariably affected, e.g. chest, eyes, lacrimal and salivary glands. The mainstay of treatment is systemic steroids.

Nasal syphilis
The congenital form may manifest as a persistent nasal discharge and fissuring of the anterior nares, and is labelled as 'snuffles'. In acquired syphilis, gummatous lesions of the nose are not uncommon. Destruction of bone and cartilage in the septum is frequent in the tertiary stage.

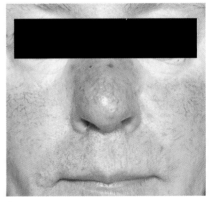

Fig. 6 **Rosacea.**

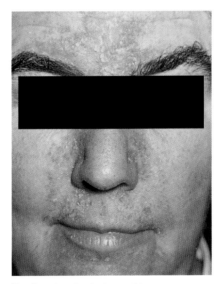

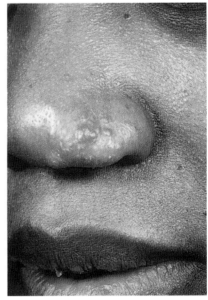

Fig. 4 **Furunculosis (boil) of the left nasal vestibule.**

Fig. 5 **Seborrhoeic dermatitis.**

Fig. 7 **Nasal sarcoidosis (lupus pernio).**

Nasal infections

■ Nasal infections can spread to the cavernous sinus.

■ Exclude neoplasia in persistent nasal ulceration.

■ In recurrent nasal furunculosis, exclude diabetes mellitus and look for a source of staphylococci.

Nasal septal pathologies and choanal atresia

Septal deflection

It is rare to find a septum that is completely in the median position. Septal deflections are most commonly due to developmental abnormalities and trauma. The deviation may involve the bony or cartilaginous regions, or both.

Clinical features

Unilateral nasal obstruction is the main complaint, although an 'S'-shaped deflection can cause bilateral symptoms. A variety of other features such as crusting, facial pain, nasal discharge and epistaxis may be attributed to deflection of the septum. Examination reveals the deflection and, frequently, an associated compensatory hypertrophy of the inferior turbinate on the opposite side (Fig. 1). Sometimes an external deformity of the nasal bridge is caused by a deviated septum (Fig. 2).

Management

Asymptomatic deflections should be left untreated. The classic operation for correcting a deviation is the *submucous resection* or SMR. This entails elevation of mucoperichondrial flaps on both sides of the septum and excision of the deformed portion. The alternative, septoplasty, is essentially a procedure which attempts to reposition the septum after the defects have been resected, with minimal removal of tissue.

Nasal haemorrhage and septal haematoma are the major complications, but are generally prevented by approximating the mucoperichondrial flaps with sutures. Packs are rarely required. Collapse of the nasal dorsum is a late feature due to excessive removal of septal cartilage (Fig. 3).

Septal haematoma

Septal haematoma is caused by nasal trauma, which can frequently be quite mild (p. 43). It is most common in children, as the mucoperichondrium is only loosely adherent to the underlying cartilage.

Clinical presentation

Severe nasal obstruction is caused by haemorrhage into the subperichondrial space (Fig. 4). Marked tenderness is not a feature unless the haematoma subsequently becomes infected. If an abscess supervenes, cartilage necrosis is inevitable and results ultimately in collapse of the nose and an ugly external deformity (saddle nose).

Management

The haematoma should be drained. This is effected either by needle aspiration, or formal incision and evacuation if the blood has clotted. Nasal packing will prevent recurrence.

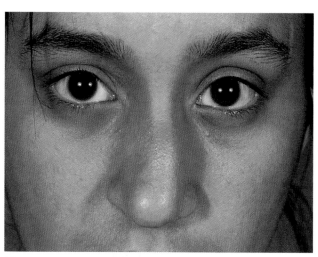

(a)

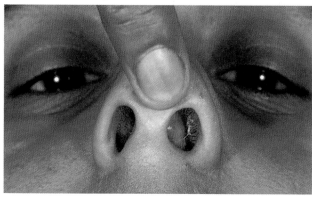

(b)

Fig. 2 **A significant external nasal deformity (a) caused by a severe deflection of the nasal septum producing almost total left nasal blockage (b).**

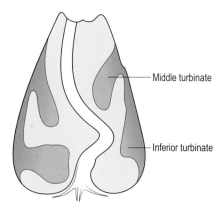

Middle turbinate

Inferior turbinate

Fig. 1 **A deflected nasal septum obstructing the left nasal airway.** The inferior turbinate has shrunk on the ipsilateral side, but has hypertrophied on the contralateral side.

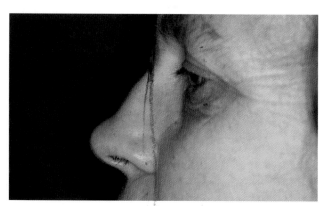

Fig. 3 **Saddle deformity.** This was due to dorsal collapse of the nose secondary to overenthusiastic removal of septal cartilage during a submucous resection for a deflected nasal septum.

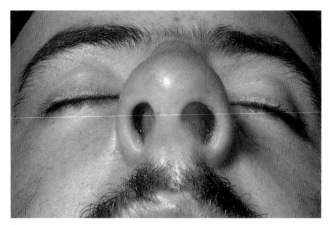

Fig. 4 **A post-traumatic septal haematoma.** Notice the thickened bulky septum encroaching on the nasal airways. The external nose is also swollen.

Antibiotics are mandatory to prevent infection and the potentially lethal complication of cavernous sinus thrombosis.

Septal perforation

There are many causes of a septal perforation, with previous septal surgery on the list (Table 1). In many cases it is not possible to implicate any specific aetiology. The majority of perforations are located in the anterior cartilaginous portion of the septum. Classically, syphilitic infection involves the more posterior bony septum.

Clinical features and management

The clinical complaints include crusting and recurrent epistaxis. Whistling respiration may also occur. It is important to elucidate the precise aetiology of the perforation if possible. Suspected neoplasia should be biopsied.

Since, in the majority of cases, no aetiological cause is apparent, treatment is symptomatic. Crusting and epistaxis may be prevented by keeping secretions soft with steam inhalations and nasal douching. Simple ointments can be applied topically to reduce crust formation. Surgical closure is possible for small to medium-sized holes, and is the treatment of choice if the septum is not atrophic. Occlusion with appropriately shaped Silastic buttons is a recent innovation.

Choanal atresia

Choanal atresia is a rare congenital abnormality due to failure of canalization of the bucconasal membrane. The natural communication between the nose and pharynx – the choana – is blocked unilaterally or bilaterally. Structurally, it is either bony or membranous.

Clinical features

Bilateral cases present at birth with severe respiratory difficulties as neonates are obligate nasal breathers and have not acquired the adult habit of mouth breathing. Unilateral choanal atresia usually presents later in life with symptoms of complete unilateral nasal blockage and mucoid discharge. At birth, the diagnosis is made by the inability to pass a soft catheter pernasally, and confirmed by the demonstration of the atretic plate with CT scanning (Fig. 5). In adults, nasal endoscopy may reveal the blocked posterior choana.

Management

Bilateral atresia is a neonatal emergency; an oral airway is inserted and fixed in position. Pernasal or transpalatal surgical approaches can be employed, depending on the precise nature of the atresia. Indwelling tubes are inserted (Fig. 6) to prevent reclosure. Regular bouginage may be necessary for many months after surgery. In unilateral cases, surgery can be delayed.

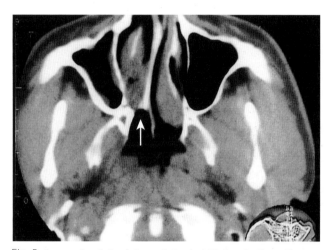

Fig. 5 **A case of unilateral choanal atresia with the atretic portion indicated.**

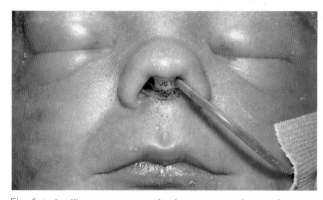

Fig. 6 **Indwelling stents are emplyed to prevent reclosure after surgery for choanal atresia.** A left-sided nasogastric tube is present for feeding.

Table 1 **Causes of septal perforation**	
Trauma	**Neoplasia**
Nasal surgery	Squamous cell carcinoma
Physical (repeated cauterization)	Malignant granuloma
Digital	Basal cell carcinoma
Infection	**Miscellaneous**
Syphilis	Chrome gases
Tuberculosis	Cocaine sniffing
	Idiopathic

Nasal septal pathologies and choanal atresia

- Septal haematoma requires urgent drainage to prevent abscess formation and cartilage necrosis.
- Asymptomatic septal deflection should be left untreated.
- Bilateral choanal atresia is a neonatal emergency.

Facial trauma

Facial trauma is often first seen during parturition, as the head diameter in the neonate is generally larger than that of the birth canal. More permanent damage can occur in varying degrees throughout life. The most severe injuries tend to be more common in adults than in children. Injury can occur to the soft tissues of the face and to the facial bones. The latter comprise the mandible, maxilla, malar complex and the nose. Extensive trauma may involve several different tissue injuries and require urgent intervention to prevent respiratory obstruction, inhalational problems and torrential haemorrhage. Most patients will require tetanus prophylaxis and antibiotic therapy.

Soft tissue trauma

The most frequent lesions encountered are lacerations. The wound should be scrubbed to avoid tattooing, and accurate skin closure is vital to prevent the need for scar revision. More severe injuries should be explored to exclude damage to deeper structures. Lost tissue, e.g. a portion of nose or ear, should be resutured. These will frequently survive due to the excellent facial blood supply.

Bony trauma

In general, only displaced fractures will require surgical correction.

Mandibular fractures

The common sites of mandibular fractures are shown in Figure 1. The weakest part of the mandible is the condylar neck; even indirect trauma may cause fractures at this site.

Clinical features

Clinically, the patient has severe trismus. Haemorrhage is usual, as is dental malocclusion if the tooth-bearing area is fractured. Bimanual palpation will reveal mobile bony fragments. X-rays will highlight the precise fracture line.

Management

In treatment, the fracture is reduced and immobilized for several weeks by wiring the upper and lower alveolar teeth together, or by miniplate stabilization.

Malar fractures

Malar fractures are common and usually follow a direct blow to the cheek bone or zygoma (Fig. 2).

Clinical features

The fracture produces a depression which may be obscured by soft tissue swelling. Palpation of the bony contours will reveal a step over the infraorbital ridge. Damage to the infraorbital nerve results in sensory loss in the cheek (Fig. 6, p. 45).

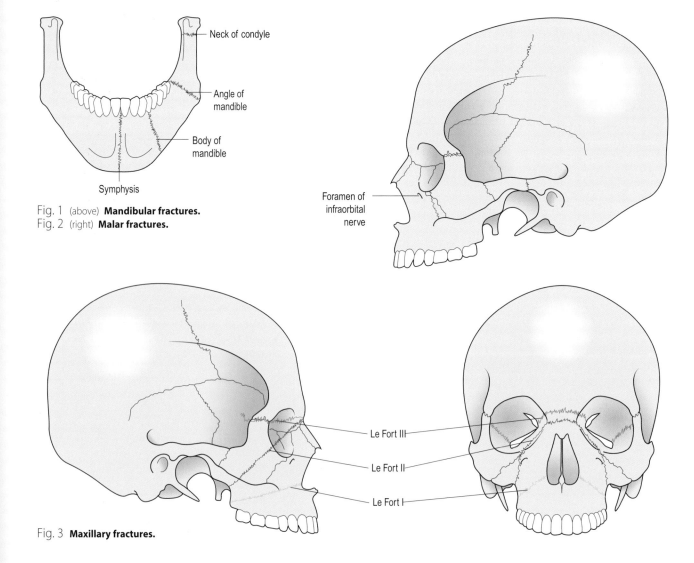

Fig. 1 (above) **Mandibular fractures.**
Fig. 2 (right) **Malar fractures.**

Neck of condyle
Angle of mandible
Body of mandible
Symphysis
Foramen of infraorbital nerve

Le Fort III
Le Fort II
Le Fort I

Fig. 3 **Maxillary fractures.**

Management

Surgical correction is performed by elevation of the depressed fragment via an incision in the temporal area. Instability after reduction will require wiring or miniplate fixation.

Maxillary fractures

A French doctor by the name of Le Fort described the three commonest fractures of the maxillary facial bone. These have been named Le Fort I, II, III fractures (Fig. 3). The maxilla provides a shock absorber function to prevent severe damage to the skull and intracranial contents. A Le Fort I fracture line passes through the inferior wall of the antrum and allows the tooth-bearing segments of the upper jaw to move in relation to the nose. A Le Fort II allows the maxilla and the nose, as a block, to move in relation to the frontal bone and zygoma. The most severe trauma produces a Le Fort III, which separates the facial bones from the skull base.

Clinical features

Severe haemorrhage and fatal airway obstruction can complicate these fractures. It is imperative to maintain the airway by holding the mandible forward. Palpation reveals bony irregularities and it is possible to show abnormal movement at the maxilla by moving the palate and alveolus while the forehead is held stationary.

Management

These fractures require reduction and splinting for several weeks. Miniplating techniques (Fig. 4) have now superseded box or halo frames for many patients.

Orbital blow-out fracture

Orbital blow-out fracture is usually caused by direct trauma which pushes the eye into the orbit, thus increasing the pressure in a relatively closed cavity. The weakest part of the cavity, the orbital floor, is fractured with extrusion of orbital contents into the maxillary antrum (Figs 5 & 6).

Clinical features

The cardinal clinical feature is limitation of eye movement due to entrapment of fibrous septa in orbital fat, or uncommonly the inferior rectus muscle. Enophthalmos is due to orbital herniation.

Management

Satisfactory management requires freeing the orbital contents and reconstruction of the floor with a sheet of Silastic or a bone graft. The fracture and prolapsed orbital contents are approached via a lower eyelid incision,

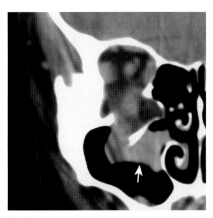

Fig. 5 **A coronal CT scan showing an extensive orbital blow-out fracture.** Notice how the soft tissue of the orbit has extruded into the roof of the maxillary antrum.

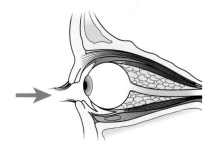

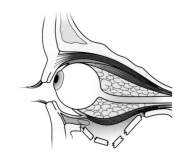

Fig. 6 **Orbital blow-out fracture.**

often combined with an endoscopic reduction via the sinus.

Nasal fractures

Nasal fractures result from either *lateral* or *frontal* forces. The former is the commonest nasal injury encountered, and lateral displacements can be corrected immediately. If this is not practical, a delay of 7 days is usual to allow soft tissue swelling to subside and an accurate assessment of the deformity to be made. Reduction is performed under local or general anaesthetic and a plaster of Paris splint applied to hold the mobile fragments in position.

If the patient presents very late, so that bony union of the fragments has occurred, then cosmetic correction is feasible by performing a rhinoplasty.

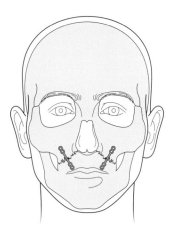

Fig. 4 **A maxillary fracture which — post reduction — is splinted using miniplating.**

Facial trauma

- Facial trauma can result in life-threatening haemorrhage, respiratory obstruction and inhalation injury.
- Most facial fractures can be diagnosed on clinical examination.
- Always examine for ocular involvement.
- Intraoral examination is mandatory.
- The infraorbital and inferior dental nerves are very commonly injured.
- Unstable fractures will require appropriate forms of splinting.
- Most nasal fractures are produced by lateral traumatic forces.
- Correction of nasal fractures should be either immediate or after the swelling has resolved at about 7–10 days.

Complications of facial trauma

The consequences of most facial trauma are comparatively minor. However, certain complications can be fatal, and even some non-life-threatening complications may lead to severe morbidity.

Clinical box
Emergency treatment will be required for:
- respiratory obstruction
- haemorrhage
- inhalational injuries.

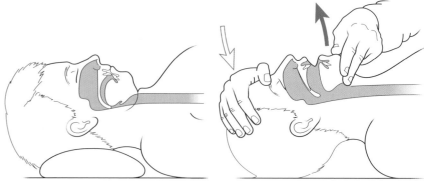

Fig. 1 **Opening the airway for resuscitation.**

Respiratory obstruction
There are multiple causes for airway obstruction, and an awareness of these may prevent a fatal outcome. Intraoral blood clots are common, but blockage due to dentures or tooth fragments must not be overlooked. Facial fractures, particularly those of the mandible and maxilla, may narrow the oropharyngeal isthmus. The tongue may cause obstruction by posterior movement of the mandible or due to traumatic swelling and oedema. In severe trauma, associated laryngotracheal injuries may be the cause.

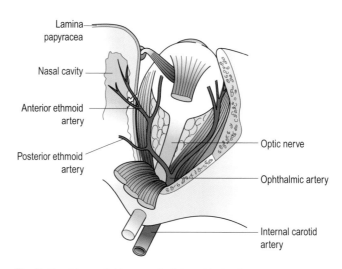

Fig. 2 **The thin medial bony wall of the orbit (lamina papyracea) is easily fractured and may tear the anterior ethmoidal artery, resulting in brisk epistaxis.**

Management
It is important to restore the airway immediately. This may be simply achieved by removing any obstructing object from the mouth or pulling the jaw forward to overcome the posterior displacement of the tongue (Fig. 1). Intubation or tracheostomy should be performed if a secure airway is not rapidly obtained.

Haemorrhage
Some degree of haemorrhage is the rule in facial trauma. Usually this settles spontaneously or can be easily controlled by direct pressure. Torrential haemorrhage may occur and is invariably due to major blood vessel damage caused by a bony fracture or sharp object. In the nose, a fracture of the lamina papyracea can tear the anterior ethmoidal artery (Fig. 2) to give brisk epistaxis (p. 48). Division of major arteries in the neck results in severe haemorrhage. Associated neck trauma can lead to bleeding from the carotid tree.

Management
Management involves immediate measures such as direct pressure to stem the flow of blood. Nasal packing may be required. Neck exploration to tie off major vessels is occasionally necessary.

Inhalation injuries
Inhalation injuries are a potentially fatal complication, especially in severe trauma with loss of consciousness. In a

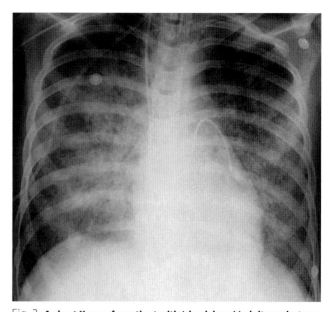

Fig. 3 **A chest X-ray of a patient with 'shock lung' (adult respiratory distress syndrome) showing the typical perihilar shadowing.** Seen also in situ are a Hickman intravenous line, a Swan–Ganz catheter and a nasogastric tube.

comatose patient, blood and gastric contents may be inhaled. If a shock lung syndrome or ARDS (adult respiratory distress syndrome) develops, the morbidity and mortality is very high (Fig. 3).

Management

Rapid institution of first-aid measures, such as ensuring the patient is in the coma position, may prevent such injuries. Intubation or tracheostomy may be necessary to prevent inhalation. In established adult respiratory distress syndrome, treatment is directed to ensuring adequate oxygenation and combating multiorgan failure.

Other complications

Cerebrospinal fluid (CSF) rhinorrhoea
A clear watery nasal discharge after facial trauma may be due to leaking of CSF. The usual site of injury is the cribriform plate or posterior wall of the frontal sinus. CSF is distinguished from normal nasal secretions in a number of ways. CSF:

- is positive to glucose testing
- produces a halo on a white cloth if mixed with blood
- contains β-transferrin on assay.

The diagnosis may be confirmed by the collection of fluorescein in the nose after injection via a lumbar puncture. More recently, high-resolution CT scanning has provided a

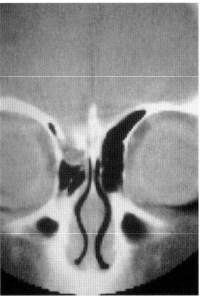

Fig. 4 **A coronal CT scan showing a traumatic fracture of the right cribriform plate with prolapse of anterior cranial fossa contents.**

very effective way of localizing fractures (Fig. 4).

Management
Some leaks will settle spontaneously with conservative measures to lower CSF pressure, such as nursing the patient upright and insertion of an epidural drain. Persistent CSF leaks may be repaired endoscopically or via a craniotomy. CSF leaks are associated with an increased risk of meningitis.

Cavernous sinus thrombosis
Cavernous sinus thrombosis is a potentially fatal complication of infected facial wounds. It is a retrograde infection, via the facial veins, resulting in an intracranial thrombosis (Fig. 5).

The condition is characterized by headaches, rigors, exophthalmos and ophthalmoplegia. High-dose parenteral antibiotics are mandatory to prevent the high mortality seen in the past.

Septal haematoma
Septal haematoma can occur as a complication of facial trauma. This condition is discussed fully on page 40.

Sensory loss
Sensory loss – producing an area of anaesthesia – is a common accompaniment of fractures of the infraorbital region with damage to the infraorbital nerve (Fig. 6). Post-traumatic anosmia is not an infrequent occurrence. Even relatively minor trauma may damage the delicate olfactory nerve filaments. Anosmia is invariable if the cribriform plate has been fractured. Unfortunately, there is no prospect of recovery.

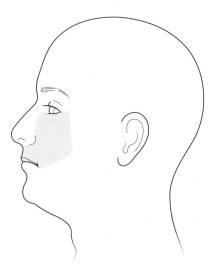

Fig. 6 **Area of sensory loss resulting from damage to the infraorbital nerve.**

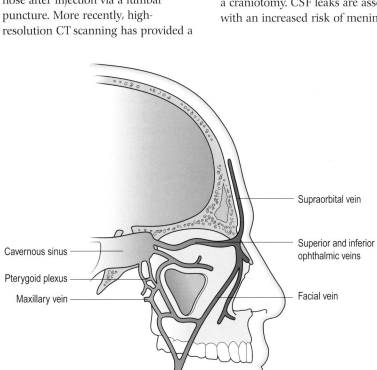

Supraorbital vein

Superior and inferior ophthalmic veins

Cavernous sinus

Pterygoid plexus

Maxillary vein

Facial vein

Fig. 5 **Cavernous sinus thrombosis.** Notice how the venous drainage of the face (via the facial and ophthalmic veins) may allow retrograde spread of infection in the facial area resulting in a thrombosis of the cavernous sinus.

> ### Complications of facial trauma
>
> - Respiratory obstruction after facial trauma may be fatal. If in difficulty, intubate or perform a tracheostomy to secure the airway.
> - Haemorrhage may be massive and fatal.
> - CSF leaks are associated with a risk of meningitis.
> - Superficial infections of the face can result in cavernous sinus thrombosis.

Facial plastic surgery

Introduction

Greater awareness and concern about facial appearance have meant an increase in the number of patients seeking corrective aesthetic facial surgery. The otolaryngologist is frequently asked about facial surgery while treating related functional problems, particularly in relation to the nose. Some patients with obvious gross disproportions are embarrassed about requesting corrective operations, while at the other end of the spectrum thera are those who overexaggerate a minor cosmetic deformity, almost to the point of obsession. It is therefore vital that adequate attention is given to the patient's psychological, as well as physical, profile to ensure they have realistic expectations of what can be performed. This is essential to avoid dissatisfaction, and sometimes the views of a psychologist and psychiatrist are useful.

Excision of facial lesions

Skin lesions are common in the face and may be sited in awkward places, e.g. the canthus of the eye or the nasal tip. Accurate preoperative diagnosis of the lesion is imperative in deciding the optimum treatment. There are now many modalities available to remove cutaneous lesions apart from excision: freezing, cautery/electrosurgery, curettage, laser and ionizing radiation. Where there is any doubt about the histology, biopsy either from the edge or via complete excision is preferable to destructive removal.

Excision of lesions should be performed with the incisions placed in the relaxed skin tensions of the face (Fig. 1). This produces the least tension on the repair and the best cosmetic scar. Larger defects which cannot be closed by simple undermining and advancement of the edges require a flap or free skin graft (Fig. 2).

Laser surgery has gained popularity recently for facial lesions and for resurfacing areas of the face. The different types of laser (wavelength) have separate applications. CO_2 lasers vaporize skin and, when combined with an oscillating beam, can precisely

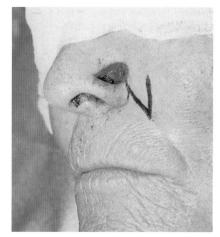

(a)

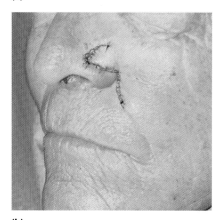

(b)

Fig. 2 **Transposition flap from nasolabial fold.**

remove tissue to a calculated depth, allowing regeneration from the adnexae (Fig. 3). Pigmented lesions, e.g. telangiectasia, will absorb the green light of an argon, KTP or pulsed diode laser, producing selective thrombosis in vessels.

Rhinoplasty

There are many variations in nasal form which can be altered by trauma or disease. Patients request rhinoplasty for a variety of reasons: females often because the nose is too large, usually with a dorsal hump (Fig. 4); males frequently because of a combination of functional and cosmetic problems, often trauma related. Deviated noses invariably have an associated septal deformity which it is essential to identify and correct at the same time as the rhinoplasty.

Most reduction rhinoplasties are performed as closed procedures, i.e. the incisions are entirely within the nasal fossa. Selected post-trauma cases

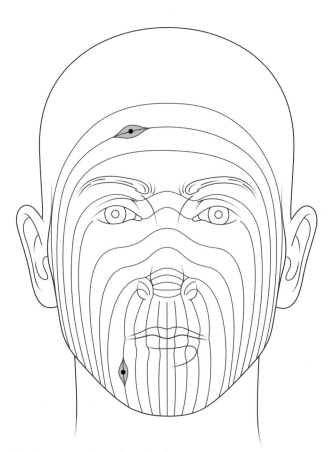

Fig. 1 **Relaxed skin tension lines for excision of facial lesions.**

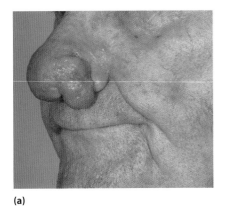

(a)

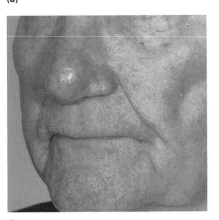

(b)

Fig. 3 **Laser skin resurfacing.**

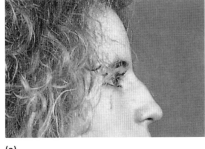

(a)

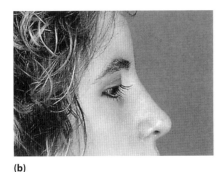

(b)

Fig. 4 **Reduction rhinoplasty.**

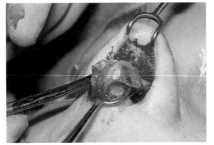

Fig. 5 **External approach rhinoplasty.**

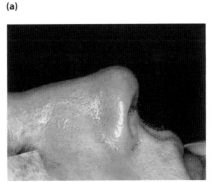

(a)

(b)

Fig. 6 **Cartilage graft augmentation of nasal saddle.**

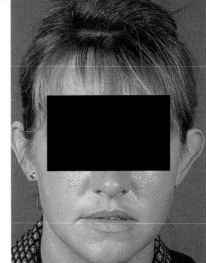

(a)

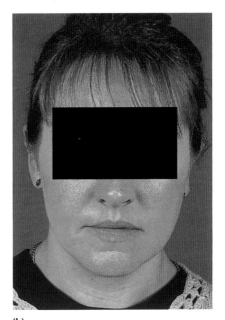

(b)

Fig. 7 **Adult otoplasty.**

and revisions may be approached by an external incision across the columella, allowing an extended range of surgical options (Figs 5 & 6).

Weak or underprojected chins should be augmented via an implant to improve the profile appearance. This often produces better balance and allows a more conservative reduction of the nose.

Otoplasty

Prominent ears are a source of ridicule for many children, and patients often feel self-conscious in adult life. The deformity is usually a combination of a deep conchal bowl and failure of the antehelix to develop. The latter, if recognized at birth, can be treated with taping over a splint within the first 5 days. Otherwise, correction is best left until just before school entry, but can be considered at any age after about three and a half years. Various techniques using cartilage scoring and sutures are employed, usually under general anaesthetic for children, and the bandages are removed at about 10 days. A sweatband is worn at night for a further 2–3 weeks. Otoplasty in an adult, particularly if it is unilateral, can be performed under local anaesthetic (Fig. 7).

> ### Facial plastic surgery
>
> ■ Biopsy is recommended if the clinical diagnosis is in doubt.
>
> ■ Gently squeeze the skin in different planes to determine the natural folds of the relaxed tension lines.
>
> ■ Refer patients to a specialist with particular interest in facial plastic surgery.

Epistaxis

For the patient, a nose bleed – even a trivial one – can often be a traumatic and frightening event. It is important to appreciate that epistaxis can be massive and rapidly fatal. The majority of epistaxes are self-limiting but it is vital to approach all cases, even minor ones, in a systematic way.

Aetiology

It is useful to divide the causes of epistaxis into local and general (Table 1). Approximately 90% of epistaxis occurs in Kiesselbach's plexus, localized at the anterior portion of the septum (Little's area; p. 30). Here a rich vascular anastomotic supply is formed by end arteries.

One of the most common local causes of epistaxis is digital trauma or nose picking, which can readily damage the delicate nasal mucosa. Another local cause is viral infection in the nose, which is frequently accompanied by nose bleeds.

Among the general causes of epistaxis, hypertension is a common feature. It does not cause epistaxis per se, but ensures continued haemorrhage once it commences. Arteriosclerosis and other cardiovascular disease also contribute to epistaxis.

Coagulation defects constitute another cause of epistaxis and may occur as a consequence of systemic disease such as leukaemia. However, certain drug groups produce a similar outcome either by design (anticoagulants) or fault (aspirin can inhibit platelet function).

Hereditary haemorrhagic telangiectasia (Osler–Weber–Rendu disease), which is characterized by abnormal capillaries, is a potent cause of recurrent epistaxis (Fig. 1). The condition can also cause haematuria,

melaena and subarachnoid or cerebral haemorrhage. All types of nasal and paranasal neoplasia may produce nasal haemorrhage, but particularly a benign vascular tumour called a juvenile angiofibroma (p. 109).

Management

Management of epistaxis involves four steps:

- initial first-aid measures
- assessment of blood loss
- evaluation of the cause
- procedures to stop continued bleeding.

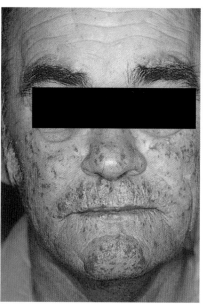

Fig. 1 **Hereditary haemorrhagic telangiectasia.** The diagnosis is obvious due to multiple skin lesions. At the time of the photograph the patient had required over 150 units of blood, and bilateral anterior ethmoidal, maxillary and external carotid ligation. Additionally he had several embolizations. Despite all these measures he still suffers from recurrent epistaxis.

First-aid measures

The nostrils should be pinched together tightly and respiration continued through the mouth. A suitable container placed under the chin will catch any blood. The subject should sit upright to lower the blood pressure and lean forward so as not to swallow blood. These manoeuvres comprise 'Trotter's method' for the control of epistaxis. It is useless to compress the bony root of the nose (Fig. 2).

If a patient presents with epistaxis in which first-aid measures have failed, and in which simple cauterization (see below) does not prevent further bleeding, hospital admission will be required for assessment of blood loss, and to identify the cause of bleeding and control the continued epistaxis.

Assessment of blood loss

A clinical assessment is made by recording the pulse and blood pressure. It is vital to appreciate that in the young an adequate blood pressure may be maintained by a rising pulse rate, but decompensation may be sudden. Other signs of shock should be looked for, e.g. pallor and sweating. An intravenous line should be inserted, blood taken for cross-matching and a suitable plasma expander commenced. A baseline haemoglobin, full blood count and clotting screen should also be requested.

Evaluation of cause

If the epistaxis has abated it is frequently possible to visualize the site of bleeding. This is particularly true of bleeding points in Little's area. Examination may reveal the presence of a foreign body or a neoplastic growth. Should blood clots prevent an

Table 1 **Aetiology of epistaxis**	
Type	**Causes**
Local	Idiopathic*
	Infection
	Trauma*
	Neoplasia
	Foreign body
General	Hypertension
	Drugs (anticoagulants)
	Blood diseases (leukaemia)
	Hereditary haemorrhagic telangiectasia

* Most common causes of epistaxis.

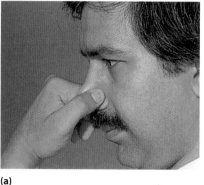

(a)   (b)

Fig. 2 **Manual compression of the nose.** The technique is performed correctly in (a). No benefit is gained by attempting to apply pressure over the bony nasal pyramid (b).

adequate view, the nose should be cleared by blowing. Topical anaesthesia produced by inserting cotton wool soaked in an appropriate solution will allow a greater degree of manipulation. It is wise to wear gloves, eye protectors and a gown. Suction aspiration should be to hand. If possible, an attempt should be made to determine whether the haemorrhage is arising from above the middle turbinate (internal carotid territory) or below (external carotid territory). Primary haematological disoders may be diagnosed from blood test results.

Controlling the bleeding

The precise method employed to control epistaxis is dependent on whether the bleeding has temporarily ceased, and the suspected site of haemorrhage. An obvious site of bleeding may be noted, or indicated by a surface blood clot. This may be easily dealt with by cauterization after anaesthetizing the nasal mucosa. A silver nitrate stick application is the simplest method of cauterization, but electrocautery may be employed.

A nasal pack will be required if no clear bleeding point is discernible. Traditionally the pack consists of ribbon gauze impregnated with bismuth iodoform paraffin paste (BIPP). The nose must be cleared of clots prior to insertion and the pack built up in layers starting in the floor (Fig. 3). It is important to appreciate that, in an adult, the distance between the anterior nares and posterior choanae is upwards of 6 cm. An inflatable balloon tamponade can be used as an alternative method of packing (Fig. 4), or microporous sponges.

Continued haemorrhage despite an anterior pack is probably due to bleeding from the posteriorly placed branches of the sphenopalatine artery and may require insertion of a postnasal pack. Specialized nasal inserts with a double balloon will allow pressure to be exerted in both the postnasal and anterior nasal spaces (Fig. 4). A formal gauze postnasal pack usually requires a general anaesthetic for insertion. Its dimensions should be similar to the distal phalanx of the patients thumb, as this compares favourably with the size of the postnasal space.

Antibiotic cover is mandatory if a postnasal pack is in situ, or if an anterior pack is left longer than 48 hours. In the elderly, it is not unusual for an acute confusional state to develop due to iodine toxicity from BIPP packs. Mild hypoxia is not uncommon after the nose is packed, and this may work synergistically with iodine toxicity.

If, despite these measures, epistaxis continues or recurs then a formal examination under anaesthetic will be needed. An obvious bleeding point may be seen endoscopically and controlled by diathermy. If not, arterial ligation of the sphenopalatine artery endoscopically, or ligation of the maxillary artery by an approach via the maxillary antrum, may be necessary. Rarely, the external carotid artery in the neck may be ligated.

In some cases, where expertise is available, embolization of the bleeding vessel can be performed under radiological control. Small pieces of gelfoam are employed to block the offending vessels.

General measures

The patient is nursed in the upright position. However, if in shock, circulation to the brain can be maintained by the head-down, feet-up posture. Carefully considered use of sedatives is useful in counteracting the anxiety which can

result in a rise of blood pressure. Any hypertensive tendency will require suitable drug therapy. Specific aetiological causes such as leukaemia or neoplasia will require management once the epistaxis is controlled.

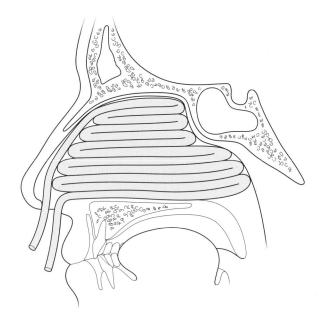

Fig. 3 **Anterior nasal packing employing BIPP.**

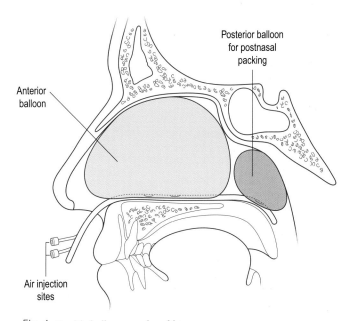

Fig. 4 **Double balloon nasal packing.**

> ### Epistaxis
>
> - Epistaxis can kill.
> - Most epistaxis is due to bleeding from Little's area and is easily managed by cauterization under local anaesthesia.
> - Inflatable balloons are more convenient to insert and less traumatic to the nasal mucosa than ribbon gauze packs.
> - Always consider both local and general pathologies in the aetiology of epistaxis. Blood loss is often underestimated.
> - Keep a steady nerve.

Acute and chronic sinusitis

Definition
Sinusitis is an inflammatory process involving the lining of the paranasal sinuses.

Aetiology
The majority of sinusitis is rhinogenic in origin but dental disease, facial trauma and neoplasia may be predisposing factors. As the lining of the nose is continuous with that of the paranasal sinuses, any mechanism producing rhinitis will have the potential to cause a sinusitis. The maxillary, frontal and sphenoidal sinuses drain into the nasal fossae via the ethmoid sinuses; this is important as conditions in the ethmoids and particularly in the middle nasal meatus will dictate what occurs in the remaining dependent larger sinuses. The aetiology of the rhinitis must be treated if sinus disease is to be satisfactorily managed.

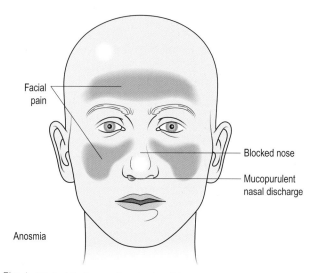

Fig. 1 **Clinical features of acute sinusitis.**

Acute sinusitis

Acute sinusitis is commonly caused by a viral rhinosinusitis. Blockage of the sinus ostia and paralysis of the mucociliary clearance mechanism causes mucus retention which, if not cleared, becomes secondarily infected by resident bacterial organisms of the nose. Any mechanical obstruction to natural airflow, such as nasal polyposis, a deflected nasal septum or turbinate hypertrophy, will also contribute to the development of infection.

The diagnosis of sinusitis is not usually difficult (Figs 1 & 2), and more than one sinus is usually involved. Facial swelling suggests complications of sinusitis, dental disease or uncommonly malignancy and therefore demands further investigation.

Treatment
Treatment consists of symptomatic relief of pain and specific therapy to overcome ostial blockage and bacterial infection. This includes:

- analgesics such as paracetamol or codeine for pain relief
- nasal drops such as oxymetazoline or ephedrine to reduce congestion of nasal mucosa
- broad-spectrum antibiotics
- steam or menthol inhalations
- aspiration of sinus contents if the above fails (Fig. 3).

Prognosis
The majority of cases of acute sinusitis resolve with medical therapy. Failure to respond suggests inadequate primary therapy or an underlying chronic sinus disease.

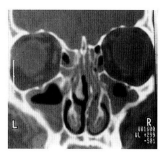

Fig. 2 **Coronal CT scan showing bilateral acute pansinusitis.** There is a fluid level in the left maxillary sinus, which if aspirated can be sent for microbiology.

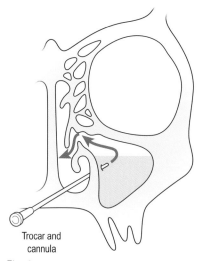

Trocar and cannula

Fig. 3 **Proof puncture.** This procedure allows aspiration and irrigation of the maxillary sinus to encourage restoration of normal mucociliary clearance when medical therapy has failed after acute infection.

Acute frontal sinusitis

Acute frontal sinusitis is a potentially serious condition because of the risk of intracranial complications, which still have a high morbidity and significant mortality (Fig. 4).

Severe frontal headache and tenderness over the sinus are usually present. CT scanning is indicated if there are suspected complications, such as orbital or intracranial involvement (Figs 5 & 6).

Treatment
Treatment of acute frontal sinus infection should involve:

- high-dose broad-spectrum antibiotics; reviewed after identifying causative organism by culture of pus
- topical vasoconstrictor nose drops to decongest the nasal mucosa and encourage normal sinus ventilation
- resolution of concomitant maxillary, ethmoidal and sphenodial sinusitis (pansinusitis) using proof puncture (Fig. 3)

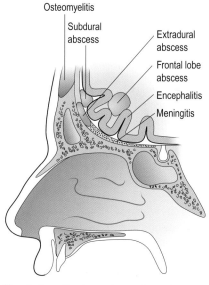

Fig. 4 **Complications of acute frontal sinusitis.**

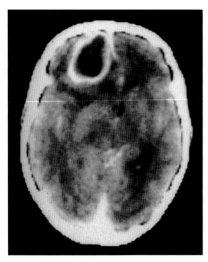

Fig. 5 **Frontal lobe abscess seen in a CT scan.**

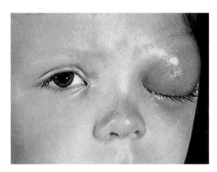

Fig. 6 **Orbital abscess due to ethmoiditis.**
Most frequently seen in children, this can also occur due to extension of acute frontal sinusitis.

■ trephination and drainage – if necessary to release the pus and culture infective material (Fig. 7).

Chronic sinusitis

Retained secretions allow a spectrum of bacteria to colonize the sinuses, further inhibiting clearance. The clinical features of chronic sinusitis include:

■ chronic purulent nasal and postnasal discharge
■ nasal block
■ facial discomfort and headaches
■ halitosis.

Expansion of an obstructed sinus is called a mucocele. This occurs in the ethmoid, the frontal and, uncommonly, in the sphenoid sinuses and requires surgery.

Treatment
With established chronic sinus disease, surgery is directed at allowing adequate drainage and removing irreversibly diseased sinus mucosa. This may involve surgery of more than

one sinus (usually the ethmoidal and maxillary). However, surgery will not cure a 'mucosal disease', e.g. allergy, and so adequate medical therapy in the form of decongestant sprays and antibiotics usually has to continue. The surgical modalities are discussed below.

Ethmoid sinus
■ *Intranasal ethmoidectomy*, often performed using an endoscope, is becoming the preferred surgical option for recurrent acute or chronic sinusitis. Via this route a physiological fenestration can be made into the maxillary sinus which in most cases will allow restoration of normal mucocillary clearance.
■ *External ethmoidectomy* involves a facial incision for access. This approach is less common now because of the increased use of endoscopes (Fig. 7).

Maxillary sinus
■ *Antrostomy* allows adequate ventilation and drainage. This is now performed via the natural ostium in the ostiomeatal complex (Fig. 8).

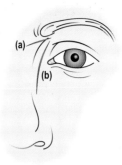

Fig. 7 **External surgical approaches to frontal ethmoid sinuses (trephination) (a) and ethmoid sinuses (b).**

■ *Caldwell–Luc operation* to allow removal of specific chronic infections, e.g. fungus, dentogenic infections, via a sublabial approach to the sinuses.

Frontal sinus
■ *Frontoethmoidectomy* – opening of the frontal sinus and floor in combination with ethmoidectomy to provide drainage into the nose. This is usually performed endoscopically.

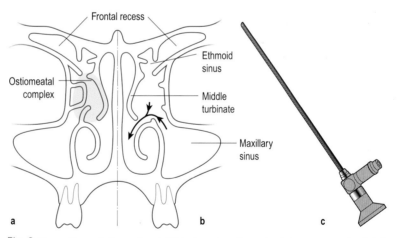

Fig. 8 **The ostiomeatal complex. (a)** This shows how the region is a common route of drainage and ventilation of the frontal, ethmoidal and maxillary sinuses. **(b)** Clearing the ostiomeatal complex allows enhanced ventilation and drainage of the dependent major paranasal sinuses. **(c)** Surgery to the ostiomeatal complex can be performed by using a rigid endoscope.

> ### Acute and chronic sinusitis
> ■ Many cases of chronic sinusitis are rhinogenic in origin.
> ■ The middle nasal meatus is the region that drains all the major paranasal sinuses, except the sphenoid.
> ■ Disease of the middle meatus and ostiomeatal complex results in pathology in the major dependent sinuses.
> ■ An acute ethmoid sinusitis is mainly a disease of children and can rapidly result in complications, e.g. orbital cellulitis.
> ■ CT scanning is invaluable in assessing the spread of acute sinus infections.

Head and neck pain I

Historically, many clinicians attributed the majority of cases of head and neck pain to sinusitis and other nasal pathologies. However, these symptoms are now known to result from a wide variety of aetiologies. Establishing a precise diagnosis is made difficult by a number of different factors. The sensory innervation of the head and neck is complex, with innumerable pain receptors in a variety of tissues. The face is also a common site for referred pain.

The management of head and neck pain demands a detailed history. A series of questions designed to elicit the cardinal clinical features of the head and neck pain will allow certain aetiologies to be unmasked (Table 1). The nature of the pain provides vital clues to possible aetiologies. Throbbing pain is usually vascular in origin due either to changes seen in migraine or to the enchanced vascularity in acute sinusitis. Sharp stabbing pains are characteristic of neuralgias, e.g. trigeminal. The position of the head, e.g. as in stooping, tends to aggravate vascular pain due to venous engorgement and is a particular feature of frontal sinusitis. Visual disturbances of a vascular origin are seen commonly in migraine, although they may also be due to optic neuritis. Any specific alteration of sensation such as numbness or hypoaesthesia associated with pain is highly suggestive of neoplastic infiltration of nervous tissue. Hence, the importance of testing for facial sensation to exclude sensory involvement.

Headaches

Headaches are a frequent complaint. Tension type headaches are the most common. Three other clinical entities are recognized and all are associated with abnormalities of the vascular tree.

Tension headaches

Tension headache is a generic term that includes headaches due to stress, disturbance of pysche and muscle contraction. They are usually episodic, but chronic symptoms can occur. The pain is bilaterally sited. The patient complains of 'a tight band around the head'. No single specific form of treatment is satisfactory. Many patients benefit from counselling designed to reduce life's stresses and provide emotional

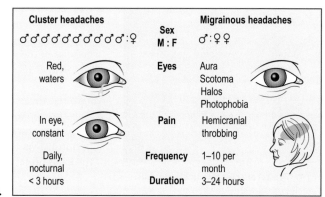

Fig. 1 **Comparison of migraine and cluster headaches.**

Cluster headaches		Migrainous headaches
♂♂♂♂♂♂♂♂♂♂:♀	Sex M : F	♂:♀♀
Red, waters	Eyes	Aura Scotoma Halos Photophobia
In eye, constant	Pain	Hemicranial throbbing
Daily, nocturnal < 3 hours	Frequency Duration	1–10 per month 3–24 hours

Table 1 **The important clinical features designed to diagnose the cause of head and neck pain**											
Clinical features	Temporo-mandibular joint dysfunction	Cervical spondylosis	Tension headaches	Migraine	Cluster headaches	Dental disease	Acute sinusitis	Neuralgias 1°	2°	Temporal arteritis	Atypical head & neck pain
Site											
1° location	Ear	Neck	Head	Hemicranium	Eye	Teeth	Over the sinus	Sensory area of trigeminal nerve V^{I-III}	Oropharynx, ear	Temple	Any site
Radiation to	Temple, cheek, neck	Ear, occiput			Nose, cheek, ear, neck	Cheek, ear		Sensory area of trigeminal nerve V^{I-III}	Oropharynx, ear	Eye	Any site
Character											
Continuous			✓ Severe constriction of head				✓			✓	
Episodic	✓	✓			✓						✓
Stabbing	✓	✓						✓	✓		✓
Throbbing				✓	✓ Severe	✓	✓			✓	✓
Aggravating factors											
Mastification	✓					✓					
Head posture		✓					✓				
Trigger zones								✓	✓		✓ Multiple
Relieving factors											Nil
Head posture		✓		✓			✓				
Analgesia	✓	✓	✓	✓	✓	✓ Partial	✓ Partial				
Darkness				✓							
Associated symptoms											
Nausea, vomiting				✓							
Visual disturbances				✓			✓ as a complication			✓	
Sensory alterations				✓					✓		
Miscellaneous		Stress, depression & muscle spasm are frequent			Lacrimation & rhinorrhoea						Many benefit from psychiatric referral

support. Headaches with a marked muscle component may resolve with simple massage. Drug therapy in the form of analgesics, antidepressants and sedatives in selected patients may provide some therapeutic gain.

Migrainous headaches

Migraines (Fig. 1) occur mainly in women and are hemicranial and paroxysmal. Prodromal eye symptoms such as halos and scotomata are not infrequent. Dilatation of intracranial vessels is the result of the disorder and in many instances can be counteracted with vasoconstrictors such as ergot preparations, beta-blockers or, for acute attacks, 5-HT agonists.

Cluster headaches

Cluster headaches (Fig. 1) are synonymous with periodic migrainous and ciliary neuralgia. The symptoms characteristically occur in the early hours, usually in clusters with periods of relief lasting several months. Prophylactic vasoconstrictors, such as those employed for migraine, are very effective.

Temporal arteritis

Temporal arteritis is characterized by a swollen and palpable superficial temporal artery. Visual defects progressing to blindness are a real danger. Pain symptoms are localized to the homolateral eye and temple. The diagnosis is made by showing a raised ESR or plasma viscosity. Urgent treatment with steroids is required on clinical grounds. If the diagnosis is in doubt, a temporal artery biopsy can be performed.

Neuralgic causes of head and neck pain

Neuralgic pains occur in the distribution of a specific nerve. The pain is invariably unilateral, episodic and extremely severe. The patient complains of 'trigger zones' which can be activated by stimuli such as touch, eating, shaving, exposure to cold winds or talking. The presence of any neurological signs (e.g. hypoasthesia) may indicate a secondary as opposed to primary neuralgia.

Primary neuralgias

Trigeminal neuralgia or tic douloureux can occur in any branch of the nerve. The ophtalmic division is most frequently involved and the pain can be triggered by combing the hair. Remission may last several months but

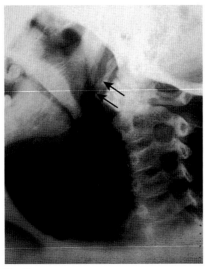

Fig. 2 **A lateral neck X-ray showing elongated styloid process.** This had resulted in glossopharyngeal neuralgia on the right side which resolved after excision of the process.

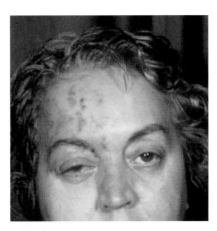

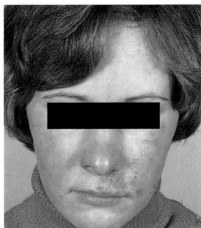

Fig. 3 **Herpes zoster infection of the opthalmic nerve** (above) **and the less frequent involvement of the maxillary nerve** (below).

relapses are frequent. Lacrimation and rhinorrhoea on ipsilateral side are common. Most cases are helped by carbamazepine. Vascular decompression by separating an aberrant blood vessel from the intracranial portion of the trigeminal nerve has also provided relief in some cases.

Glossopharyngeal neuralgia is characterized by piercing pain in the throat, which radiates to the ear. The tonsil is the trigger zone and the pain is activated by swallowing or yawning. Carbamazepine is much less effectve than in tic doulourex. Section of the glossopharyngeal nerve, either in the tonsil fossa or intracranially, has been tried with unpredictable results.

In *tympanic neuralgia* the site of pain is deep within the ear. Relief may be obtained by dividing the tympanic nerve in the middle ear.

Secondary neuralgias

Secondary neuralgias are produced by physical damage to nerves, usually as a consequence of compression or tumour infiltration.

An acoustic neuroma expanding in the cerebellopontine angle can cause pressure on the trigeminal and glossopharyngeal nerves. An elongated styloid process may give rise to symptoms of *glossopharyngeal neuralgia* by irritating the nerve as it passes the tonsil fossa (Fig. 2). Nasopharyngeal tumours can erode the skull base and cause invasion and compression of the trigeminal nerve.

Sluder's or *anterior ethmoidal neuralgia* is due to irritation of the nerve as it enters the roof of the nose. Such a situation can occur if the middle turbinate abuts the septum. Severe pain is sited at the roof of the nose and radiates to the forehead. Cocainization of the nose abolishes the symptoms and surgery to remove the turbinate septal pressure is curative.

Postherpetic neuralgia is a frequent complication of herpes zoster infection. The ophthalmic division of the trigeminal is commonly affected. Pain may continue for several months after the vesicular rash has subsided (Fig. 3).

Head and neck pain I

- In the diagnosis of head and neck pain, a clinical history is more useful than investigations.

- Tension headaches are the commonest cause of head and neck pain. The physical signs elicitable are limited or nil.

- Temporal arteritis may cause blindness. If the diagnosis is suspected, steroid treatment should be commenced on clinical grounds.

- Primary neuralgias are not accompanied by neurological signs.

- Secondary neuralgias may show evidencec of nerve deficits, and require imaging — usually MRI or CT.

Head and neck pain II

Miscellaneous causes of head and neck pain

A variety of conditions can result in referred head and neck pain (Fig. 1). Dental pathology, such as carious teeth and unerupted third molars, are common causes. Abnormalities of the cervical spine and spasm of the cervical muscles may also produce pain in the neck radiating to the ear and occiput.

Abnormalities of the temporomandibular joint

Temporomandibular joint abnormalities are a prevalent cause of facial pain. Referred otalgia is a very common symptom in this condition (p. 13), but pain may be felt in the temple and cheek. The nerve endings in the joint are stimulated by stress due to malocclusion stretching the joint capsule. The discomfort may be noted with jaw movements, e.g. chewing. Edentulous patients are frequent sufferers. Palpation may elicit pain over the joint and crepitus may be felt and heard. Treatment consists of procedures to correct the bite and muscle relaxants to relieve associated muscular spasm.

Paranasal sinus disease

Acute sinus infection produces pain localized over the involved sinus(es) and is easily diasgnosed due to constitutional upset and invariable presence of nasal symptoms. However, some cases of facial pain may be due to anatomical narrowing and localized disease in the middle meatus producing secondary sinus pathology in the maxillary, ethmoid and frontal sinuses (Fig. 2). Endoscopic surgical correction of the narrowed ostiomeatal complex will result in abolition of symptoms and restoration of normal mucosa (p. 51).

Atypical head and neck pain

A diagnosis of *atypical* head and neck pain should only be made once all potential organic causes for the symptoms have been eliminated. The patient is typically a postmenopausal woman. Extremely descriptive terms are used to explain the pain, e.g. agonizing, searing, horrifying. It is not localized to a specific site and tends to involve the whole face, head and neck. There are multiple trigger points.

The pain is so severe that the patient is incapable of continuing a normal home, social or working life. Physical examination and investigation prove negative, although many sufferers may have undergone previous surgical procedures. Earlier dental extractions are very frequent, but varying nasal operations and even intracranial nerve sections may have been performed. Unfortunately, any relief of symptom is short-lived.

Recognition of this symptom complex is essential to avoid needless operative procedures. These patients are often depressed with a disturbed pysche. Once the diagnosis has been made, a psychiatric referral is mandatory.

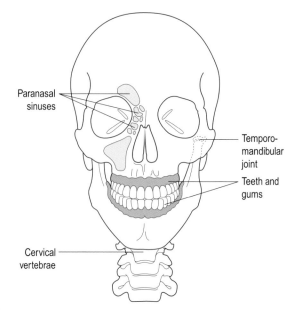

Fig. 1 **Common sites of pathology causing referred head and neck pain.**

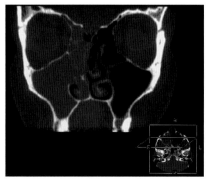

Fig. 2 **(a) CT scan showing opaque ethmoid and maxillary antra in acute sinusitis. (b) Diagrammatic representation of the importance of the ostiomeatal complex in the drainage of the major paranasal sinuses.**

(a)

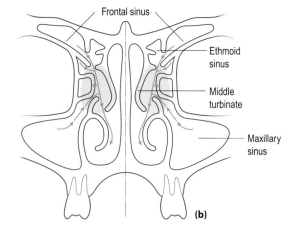

(b)

Head and neck pain II

- Acute and chronic sinusitis can result in head and neck pain.
- Many causes of head and neck pain are idiopathic.
- Referred causes of head and neck pain are very common.
- Abnormalities of the temporomandibular joint and arthritis of the cervical spine are extremely common causes of head and neck pain.
- Dental disease is a common aetiology of head and neck pain.
- Atypical head and neck pain is a diagnosis of exclusion.
- Eyestrain is a very rare cause of head and neck pain.

The Throat

Anatomy and physiology

This section will discuss the non-neoplastic diseases of the throat. The regions included in the broad term 'throat' are:

- the oral cavity
- pharynx
- larynx
- major salivary glands.

Oral cavity

The oral cavity is frequently called the mouth but, in fact, additionally comprises the anterior two-thirds of the tongue, the lips, hard palate, teeth and alveoli of the mandible and maxilla. Its major function is to provide the milieu for satisfactory mastication.

The tongue (Fig. 1) is a mass of interlacing muscle contained in a bag of cornified squamous epithelium. It contains numerous taste buds and is essential for efficient articulation, mastication and deglutition.

The teeth provide the mechanics for grinding food and are composed of enamel, dentine and cementum. The primary dentition of 20 teeth is completed by about 3 years. There are 32 teeth in the secondary (permanent) dentition commencing at about 6 years and complete by about 18 years (Fig. 2). The teeth-bearing alveoli of the maxilla are intimately related to the maxillary sinus. Occasionally the roots of the teeth may rest within the sinus cavity and lead to sinusitis secondary to dental disease.

As food is masticated it is mixed with saliva and formed into a bolus which is swallowed after the soft palate has occluded the nasopharynx from the oropharynx. This is the oral phase of deglutition (first stage) and is voluntary.

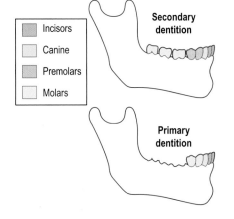

Fig. 1 **Anatomy of the tongue.**

(labels: Epiglottis; Palatine tonsil; Posterior one-third of tongue (lingual tonsil); Circumvallate papillae; Filiform papillae)

Pharynx

For clinical purposes the pharynx is divided into three regions:

- nasopharynx
- oropharynx
- hypopharynx.

It stretches from the base of the skull above to the cricopharyngeal sphincter below. The oropharynx and hypopharynx, although primarily concerned with swallowing, are so closely related to the laryngeal inlet that pathology in these areas may cause symptoms and signs in adjacent regions. The important clinical structures in each part of the pharynx are shown in Figure 3.

The pharyngeal phase of swallowing (second stage) is initiated when the bolus of food hits the posterior pharayngeal wall. The soft palate occludes the nasopharynx, the larynx is elevated and the epiglottis falls back. The last two manoeuvres protect the laryngeal inlet. Once the food enters the oesophagus it is propelled onwards by involuntary peristaltic waves (third stage).

Fig. 2 (right) **Primary and secondary dentition.** In the completed primary dentition, each one-quarter jaw contains five teeth. In the completed secondary dentition, each one-quarter jaw contains eight teeth.

(legend: Incisors; Canine; Premolars; Molars. Labels: Secondary dentition; Primary dentition)

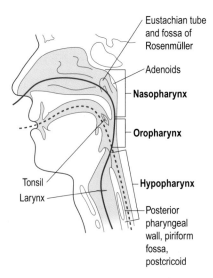

(labels: Eustachian tube and fossa of Rosenmüller; Adenoids; **Nasopharynx**; **Oropharynx**; **Hypopharynx**; Tonsil; Larynx; Posterior pharyngeal wall, piriform fossa, postcricoid)

Notice the crossover between the upper airway (–) and upper food passages (---)

Fig. 3 **The three regions of the pharynx.**

Larynx

The primary function of the larynx is to protect the tracheobronchial tree. Through evolution it has developed the secondary function of voice production. It has a rigid skeleton consisting of several cartilaginous structures (Fig. 4). The most prominent of these is the thyroid cartilage, which inferiorly articulates with the cricoid cartilage. The flap-like epiglottis is attached to the thyroid cartilage and occludes the laryngeal inlet on contraction of the aryepiglottic muscles. The cricothyroid membrane provides a suitable site through which the airway can be maintained in an emergency (see p. 68).

For descriptive purposes the larynx is subdivided into three parts:

- glottis
- supraglottis
- subglottis.

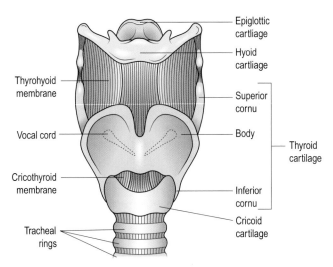

Fig. 4 **The cartilages forming the laryngeal framework.**

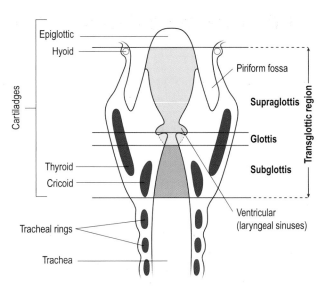

Fig. 5 **Coronal section of the larynx showing three major regional subdivisions.**

The glottis is the space between the vocal cords. The posterior third of the vocal cord is the cartilaginous arytenoids and the anterior two-thirds is membranous. The supraglottis extends from the ventricular sinus to the hyoid. The subglottis stretches from 1 cm below the glottis to the lower border of the cricoid. Food and saliva are prevented from entering the lower respiratory tract by the sphincteric action of the true and false cords. Additionally, during swallowing, the larynx is elevated pari passu with the hyoid bone so as to rest under the tongue. Food then passes into the lateral recesses (piriform sinuses) rather than in the midline. The epiglottis falls back as a part of this protective mechanism.

Voice production

The larynx also provides the basic phonatory sound upon which a voice can be produced. Adduction of the vocal cords produces a constricted area where the air pressure is reduced as it passes from the lungs to the pharynx (Bernouilli's phenomenon). The vocal cord mucosa is consequently sucked together, producing a rise in the subglottic pressure which forces the cords apart again. This cycle is repeated to produce vibration and hence sound. Volume changes are effected by alteration of the subglottic pressure. Pitch alterations occur by modifying vocal cord length and tension. The quality of the raw basic laryngeal phonatory sound is further altered by the resonating cavities of the pharynx, mouth and nose. Speech is ultimately produced by the interaction of the articulators (teeth, tongue, lips) on this phonatory sound.

Salivary glands

For clinical purposes there are three pairs of salivary glands:

- parotids
- submandibular glands
- sublingual glands.

The parotids produce a mainly serous saliva, and the submandibular glands secrete a seromucinous fluid. The parotid duct opens into the buccal sulcus opposite the second upper molar tooth. The submandibular duct opens into the floor of the mouth just lateral to the frenulum of the tongue. The sublingual glands open by multiple small ducts into the submandibular ducts and floor of the mouth. In addition, there are numerous minor salivary glands located throughout the oral cavity and pharynx. The functions of the salivary glands are related to the properties and volume of saliva (Table 1).

Lymphatic drainage

Lymph nodes in the head and neck provide a barrier to the spread of disease, either inflammatory or neoplastic. Enlargement either implies primary disease of the nodes or is secondary to pathology in the head and neck, but less commonly from

Table 1 **Functions of the saliva**
Lubricates food
Facilitates mastication and deglutition
Assists articulation
Essential for taste
Maintains oral hygiene
Protective role (contains IgA)
Commencement of digestion

sites below the clavicle. It is essential to palpate the neck in a systematic fashion so that no area is missed.

Nerve supply

The pharynx is supplied by nerve branches from the pharyngeal plexus. The laryngeal muscles, except for the cricothyroid, are innervated by the recurrent laryngeal nerve. The cricothyroid is supplied by branch of the superior laryngeal nerve. Sensation to the subglottis and glottis is from the recurrent laryngeal nerve, and the supraglottis from the superior laryngeal nerve.

In the oral cavity, ordinary sensation and the muscles of mastication are supplied by the trigeminal nerve. The tongue muscles are innervated by the hypoglossal nerve. Taste to the anterior two-thirds of the tongue is via the chorda tympani nerve which runs in the lingual nerve and via the glossopharyngeal nerve for the posterior one-third and the pharyngeal wall.

Anatomy and physiology

- Disease in either the oropharynx, hypopharynx or larynx may cause problems in adjacent structures.

- The functions of the larynx are protection of the lower respiratory tract, phonation and Valsalva.

- Lymph nodes in the neck can become involved in primary and secondary pathologies.

- An emergency airway can be maintained through the cricothyroid membrane.

Symptoms, signs and examination

The importance of a full and accurate history as an aid to diagnosis cannot be overemphasized. Direct questioning related to specific areas in the throat is essential, and smoking habits and alcohol intake must be assessed.

Symptoms and signs

Oral cavity

The major signs and symptoms of oral disease include:

- pain
- masses
- ulceration
- haemorrhage
- halitosis
- discoloration.

Pain

Dental disease is the commonest cause of pain in the oral cavity. Carious teeth are tender if subjected to temperature changes and on chewing. Periodontal disease can cause pain on tooth brushing and is associated with halitosis due to accumulation of decaying food debris. Dentures may cause pain if improperly sized, or if they provide an abnormal bite. Atrophy of the teeth-bearing alveolar ridges may result in dentures causing pain, and is commonly seen in the elderly. Maxillary sinusitis may result in toothache if a tooth root is projecting into the sinus mucosa (Fig. 1). Pain due to malignant disease is severe and constant, and invariably leads to some degree of dysphagia.

Oral masses

Any complaint of a lump requires palpation of the site, even if a lesion is not visible. Virtually all lumps require biopsy to exclude cancer. Tongue masses are nearly always neoplastic. One exception is the rare, median rhomboid glossitis which presents as a red area on the dorsum of the tongue and is benign (p. 83).

Blockage of a duct of the sublingual salivary gland may give rise to a cystic lesion called a ranula in the floor of the mouth. An exostosis of the hard palate, 'torus palatinus', has a typical position in the midline and is hard to palpation (Fig. 2).

Ulceration and haemorrhage

Persistent ulcers should be considered malignant unless proven otherwise. Recurrent painful ulcers in varying sites in the oral cavity are due to aphthous ulceration. Other causes include trauma, lichen planus, herpes and Vincent's angina. All non-healing ulcers should be biopsied.

Haemorrhage is frequently due to gum disease secondary to dental caries. However, malignancy or a bleeding diathesis may be the underlying pathology.

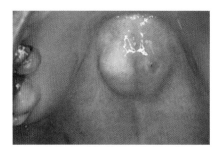

Fig. 2 **The torus palatinus is an osteoma of the hard palate, usually located in the midline.**

Halitosis (bad breath)

Poor dental hygiene is the main cause of halitosis. Decaying food debris between the teeth and in mucosal pockets in the gums are potent causes. Intake of alcohol, ingestion of garlic and use of tobacco will also give rise to a foul breath. Reflux oesophagitis and postnasal drip from chronic sinusitis may result in halitosis. Intraoral and oropharyngeal malignant disease produces a very potent offensive smell.

Discoloration

White patches (leukoplakia) and red patches (erythroplakia) have potential for malignant transformation if the cause is not removed.

Pharynx

The precise symptoms are dependent on which region of the pharynx is primarily involved. The majority of pathologies in the oropharynx and hypopharynx, either inflammatory or neoplastic, will lead to some degree of dysphagia (p. 76) (Fig. 3). Deafness may occur due to obstruction of the Eustachian tube with nasopharyngeal pathologies. Progressive nasal obstruction and epistaxis with otological symptoms should alert the clinician to nasopharyngeal malignancy. Large oropharyngeal masses may cause a voice change ('hot potato voice') and respiratory obstruction.

The alteration in voice in hypopharyngeal neoplasia is due either to direct infiltration of the larynx, or by involvement of the recurrent laryngeal nerve with development of vocal cord palsy. Secondary nodal neck masses

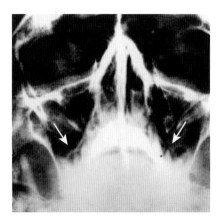

Fig. 1 **X-ray showing identation of tooth roots in the maxillary antra.**

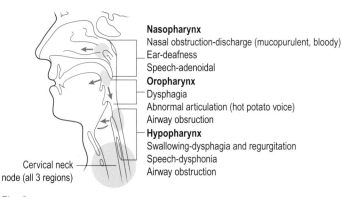

Nasopharynx
Nasal obstruction-discharge (mucopurulent, bloody)
Ear-deafness
Speech-adenoidal
Oropharynx
Dysphagia
Abnormal articulation (hot potato voice)
Airway obsruction
Hypopharynx
Swallowing-dysphagia and regurgitation
Speech-dysphonia
Airway obstruction

Cervical neck node (all 3 regions)

Fig. 3 **Symptoms of disease in the three regions of the pharynx.**

are very frequent with pharyngeal neoplasia and may be the presenting feature. Pain in pharyngeal disease may be localized to the throat, but is more usually referred to the ear.

Larynx

An alteration in voice (dysphonia) is the predominant symptom in laryngeal pathology. Respiratory difficulties usually occur late. Pain, difficulty in swallowing (dysphagia) or a lump in the neck in association with dysphonia may represent laryngeal malignancy. Aspiration of solids and liquids *may* occur with an incompetent larynx due to vocal cord paralysis, but is invariable in neurological disease producing sensory loss of the supraglottis.

Salivary glands

Pain and swelling are the two cardinal symptoms of pathology in the major salivary glands. Characteristics of the pain may lead to a specific diagnosis. If associated with mastication and some temporary swelling of the gland, particularly the submandibular, it may be due to an obstructive lesion in the salivary ducts. Continuous pain of increasing severity should heighten the suspicion of malignant disease.

A permanent enlargement of the salivary gland is neoplastic unless proven to the contrary. Sjögren's syndrome may produce swelling of one or all of the major salivary glands. Certain endocrine disease (e.g. myxoedema) and drugs (e.g. oral hypoglycaemics) may cause salivary gland hypertrophy. A weakness of the facial nerve in parotid gland disease signifies malignancy.

Neck lumps

Persistent neck lumps should be investigated. This should include fine needle aspirate cytology (FNAC), with ultrasound guidance if available. A full examination of the upper air and food passages should be carried out and biopsies taken if malignancy is suspected.

Examination

With experience it is possible to view the oral cavity and all parts of the pharynx and larynx using good illumination, tongue depressors and mirrors. These techniques are best learnt under supervision. Increasingly, laryngopharyngeal examination is

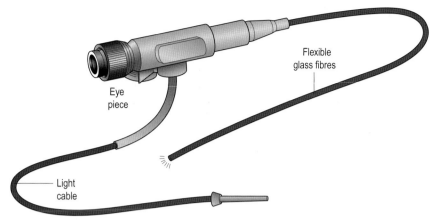

Fig. 4 **Flexible rhinolaryngoscope.** Allows examination of the nose, nasopharynx, oropharynx, larynx and hypopharynx.

carried out using a fibreoptic nasal endoscope (Fig. 4). Palpation plays a vital role in a full evaluation. Frequently a lesion may be more easily felt than visualized, and its limits readily defined. Neck palpation is essential in all cases of head and neck neoplasia.

Imaging

The value of plain radiology of the oral cavity is limited to viewing dental disease. Otherwise, CT or MRI scanning is superior. However, lateral X-rays of the pharynx are useful, and may show evidence of abnormal shadowing. Contrast swallow studies may provide information on hypopharyngeal and oesophageal pathology (Fig. 5). A variety of radiological investigations of the salivary glands are available and are selected according to the suspected pathology (Table 1).

Table 1 **Imaging techniques available in salivary gland pathology**	
Suspected pathology	**Imaging mode**
Submandibular gland calculi	Plain X-ray/ultrasound scan
Sialectasis	Sialography
Parotid calculi	CT scan/ultrasound scan
Neoplasia	MRI/CT
Autoimmune disease	Radioisotopes

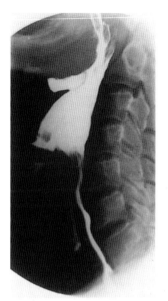

Fig. 5 **A barium swallow showing a large filling defect in the pharyngo-oesophageal region.**

Biopsy

Any persistent mass or swelling should be biopsied. In the oral cavity this may be possible with simple local anaesthesia. Masses sited in the pharynx frequently require full assessment under a general anaesthetic, and special instrumentation is required for biopsy. All laryngeal masses require biopsy. Swellings of a major salivary gland can be biopsied by fine needle aspiration, which can readily be performed as an outpatient procedure. Excision biopsies are required in all other circumstances.

Symptoms, signs and examination

- Infective and neoplastic lesions of the upper air and food passages may present as enlarged neck glands.
- All lumps should be palpated to assess their dimensions, consistency and fixity.
- All parts of the throat can be visualized on an outpatient basis.
- Contrast studies are required in cases of hypopharyngeal or oesophageal pathology.

Dysphonia — Organic causes

Voice changes are often loosely described as hoarseness, but it is preferable to use the terms *aphonia* and *dysphonia*. Aphonia should be reserved for cases with no voice or a mere whisper. Dysphonia describes an alteration in the quality of the voice. Most cases of sudden aphonia are psychogenic in origin. Laryngeal disorders can present as dysphonia which may progress to stridor (p. 64). Organic causes of dysphonia may be broadly classified as in Table 1 and are discussed below. Non-organic dysphonia is considered on pages 62–63.

Inflammatory laryngeal lesions
Acute laryngitis
Acute laryngitis is very common and frequently associated with an upper respiratory tract infection. It may also be non-infective, occurring after vocal abuse, e.g. shouting. There is invariably some pain in the throat. Resolution is spontaneous, although a degree of symptomatic relief is produced by steam inhalations and voice rest. If symptoms continue for more than 4 weeks, referral to an ENT specialist is mandatory.

Polyps and foreign bodies
Unilateral inflammatory polyps are not uncommon (Fig. 1). The history is similar to acute laryngitis, but resolution of hoarseness cannot occur until the polyp is removed under microlaryngoscopic control. Foreign bodies may only irritate the larynx to produce dysphonia (p. 84), but if lodged in the glottis may result in life-threatening respiratory obstruction. Inhalation of fumes, whether from tobacco, smoke or chemicals, may result in acute dysphonia. All inflammatory lesions, either infection

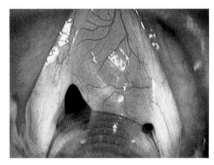

Fig. 1 **A large gelatinous polyp arising from the right vocal cord.**

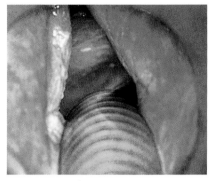

Fig. 2 **Chronic hyperplastic laryngitis.** The white appearance is leukoplakia.

or traumatic, may produce a sufficient degree of oedema to cause respiratory embarrassment.

Chronic laryngitis
Chronic dysphonia is frequently the end result of chronic laryngitis. This entitiy is produced by the long-term synergistic effect to continuing vocal abuse, alcohol ingestion and inhalation of tobacco smoke and other atmospheric pollutants. The respiratory epithelium of the larynx is replaced through metaplasia with a keratinizing squamous lining. The alteration is reflected in the macroscopic appearance of the larynx to show hypertrophic epithelium and leukoplakia (Fig. 2). Such an appearance may herald neoplastic change, so biopsy is mandatory. If neoplasia has been excluded, management is directed to avoiding known aetiological factors.

Neoplastic lesions
Neoplastic lesions causing dysphonia are discussed later in this text.

Neurological lesions
Neurological lesions may be of central or peripheral origin. Central pathologies include pseudobulbar palsy, cerebral palsy and multiple sclerosis. Peripheral pathologies include myasthenia gravis, motor neurone disease and lesions affecting the vagus and recurrent laryngeal nerves. With most peripheral causes, there will be dysarthrophonia secondary to a vocal cord paralysis.

Once a vocal cord palsy has been diagnosed and any local laryngeal pathology excluded, a systematic approach is required to determine the aetiology. This is most easily done by

considering the course of the vagus and recurrent laryngeal nerves. Because of its longer route, the left recurrent laryngeal nerve is more frequently involved by pathology (Fig. 3). On the left this will be from the cranium via the skull base, neck and thorax back to the larynx; on the right its terminates in the neck. One of the commonest causes of vocal cord palsy is primary malignant disease in the chest, with hilar involvement causing recurrent nerve deficits. Inspection of the neck may reveal the scar of previous surgery, e.g. carotid endarterectomy or thyroid surgery (Fig. 4). Unilateral vocal cord palsy, where history and examination do not reveal a cause, should therefore have CT imaging from brain stem to chest.

Spasmodic dysphonia
Spasmodic dysphonia is primarily a neurogenic disorder, although a small percentage of cases may be psychogenic in origin. The most common form is characterized by gross hyperadduction of the true and false vocal cords. The voice is distinctive and variously described as 'strained' or 'strangled'. However, during singing, crying and laughing, the voice may be normal. In some patients, the onset of symptoms is related to a major life event, e.g. bereavement, family conflicts or road accidents.

Conventional speech therapy techniques are beneficial in treating those cases of psychogenic origin, but have litle effect on those of neurogenic aetiology. Treatment involves regular injections of botulinum toxin into the vocal folds to abolish neuromuscular transmission at the motor end plate.

Table 1	**Organic causes of dysphonia**
Type	**Cause**
Inflamamtory	Acute laryngitis (infective), chronic laryngitis
Neoplasia	Carcinoma larynx, respiratory papillomata
Neurological	Myasthenia gravis, carcinoma lung/breast, post thyroidectomy, spasmodic dysphonia
Systemic	Hypothyroidism, rheumatoid arthritis

Systemic causes

A number of systemic conditions can produce dysphonia. these include the following:

- *Hypothyroidism* can produce chronic oedema of the vocal cords. It is improved by appropriate medical therapy.
- *Angioneurotic oedema*, a manifestation of a type I allergic response, can cause laryngeal oedema which initially produces dysphonia, but may progress rapidly to respiratory obstruction.

- *Rheumatoid arthritis* can result in fixation of the cricoarytenoid joint, and vocal cord immobility. Such patients invariably have severe involvement of the small joints in the hands and feet.

Management

The direction of investigation will be determined by the clinical history and physical signs. Treatment policies are then directed at abolishing or reducing the aetiological factors.

In many cases of unilateral cord palsy, no obvious aetiology is uncovered, despite extensive investigations. Such cases are eventually labelled idiopathic. Some recover spontaneously (which may take up to 12 months) or become asymptomatic as the contralateral mobile vocal cord compensates. If compensation in unilateral cord palsy is inadequate, then a medialization procedure may be beneficial. This involves techniques to medialize the palsied cord so that the

mobile cord is more easily able to effect approximation (Fig. 5).

Patients with terminal disease, e.g. carcinoma of the lung and breast, should have a medialization procedure immediately to ameliorate the distressing symptoms of dysphonia and frequently associated aspiration.

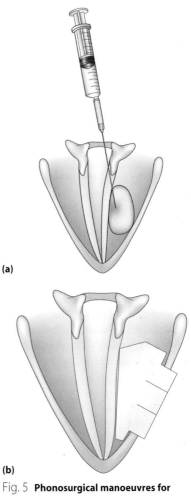

(a)

(b)

Fig. 5 **Phonosurgical manoeuvres for medializing a paralysed vocal fold.**
(a) Injection of collagen, Silastic or fat to bulk out the vocal cord. **(b)** Placement of appropriate tissue, e.g. synthetic bone or Silastic, as an implant.

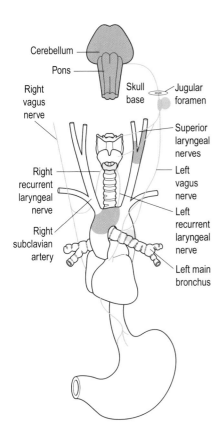

Fig. 3 **The course of the right and left vagus nerve and some of the lesions that may result in vocal cord paralysis.**

	Central lesions Cerebrovascular accident, Guillain–Barré syndrome, head injury, multiple sclerosis
	Peripheral lesions Glomus jugulare, nasopharyngeal cancer
	Carotid surgery
	Thyroid surgery, laryngeal trauma
	Carcinoma of the bronchus
	Cardiothoracic and oesophageal surgery
	Idiopathic causes Virus infection (glandular fever)

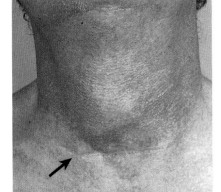

Fig. 4 **Scar due to skin incision for thyroidectomy.** The operation resulted in bilateral vocal cord paralysis due to recurrent laryngeal nerve injuries.

Dysphonia – organic causes

- Should acute dysphonia not resolve within 4 weeks, ENT referral is mandatory to exclude neoplasia.
- All cases of chronic dysphonia should be referred for laryngeal examination to exclude neoplasia.
- Avoidance of trauma (tobacco, voice abuse) will hasten resolution of acute dysphonia and improve chronic laryngitis.
- In children, acute onset dysphonia, if due to inflammatory laryngeal lesions, can rapidly lead to total respiratory obstruction.
- All vocal cord palsies with a macroscopically normal cord appearance should have a chest X-ray to exclude primary lung malignancy. If this is normal then a CT scan is required to image the course of the vagus and recurrent laryngeal nerve.

Dysphonia — Non-organic causes

Dysphonia from non-organic causes may have a psychogenic or habitual aetiology. There is no organic deficit that prevents normal function, but specific laryngeal pathology may develop secondary to misuse or abuse of the voice. Table 1 illustrates the classification of non-organic voice disorders. All age groups, from the very young to the elderly, may be affected.

Habitual dysphonias

In patients with habitual, or 'hyperkinetic', dysphonia the voice quality is frequently related to the presence of emotional stress. Most cases reveal long-term poor voice quality of gradual onset, which is generally worse after a period of talking. These features do not occur in psychogenic voice disorders. The habitual dysphonic uses incorrect patterns in voice production which may be amenable to therapy. However, prolonged habitual misuse and abuse of the vocal folds can lead to secondary organic changes. These changes may be reversible by suitable re-education, but in some instances will require surgical intervention.

Vocal abuse is caused by hyperadduction of the vocal cords and can lead to varying degrees of secondary pathology, e.g. acute inflammation, vocal cord oedema, vocal cord nodules, chronic inflammation and contact ulcers. These conditions are more common in women and children than men.

Acute non-infective laryngitis

Laryngitis can occur after an episode of aggressive singing, shouting or screaming. The basis is an emotional need to vocalize strenuously. The cords are reddened and mild oedema may

be present. On occasions, submucosal haemorrhages may occur in the vocal cords. Treatment is directed at allowing the acute inflammation to resolve and correcting any underlying vocal habits to prevent recurrence.

Vocal cord nodules

Nodules are common in male children and adult women, particularly in personalities who vocalize aggressively. The extreme vocal abuse in pop singing can also result in vocal nodules.

The nodule is located at the junction of the anterior and middle third of the vocal cord (Fig. 1). This is the area of maximum trauma at higher pitch levels seen in activities such as screaming and singing. The dysphonia is breathy and husky with a low pitch quality due to the mass loading of the vocal cords and their inability to close satisfactorily.

With suitable voice therapy directed at reducing stress and teaching normal vocal production, the majority of vocal cord nodules either resolve or are greatly improved. Only in rare instances is microlaryngoscopic excision required.

Vocal cord oedema and polyps

Oedema of the vocal cords is usually symmetrical and affects the whole length of the cord. It is due to accumulation of fluid in the subepithelial space of Reinke and is called 'Reinke's oedema'. Localization of the oedema to a circumscribed site will produce a polyp, usually sited in the anterior third of the vocal cord.

Mild oedema of the cords may resolve with improvement in the voice. More severe forms, such as Reinke's, are best treated by microsurgical removal of oedematous tissue, preserving the overlying mucosa (Fig. 2). Voice therapy should be

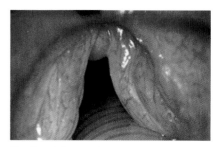
Fig. 2 **Reinke's oedema causing swelling of both vocal cords.** There is also a vocal cord polyp in the subglottis anteriorly.

instituted to correct any vocal abuse. Polyps always require surgical excision and histological analysis.

Chronic non-infective laryngitis

Epithelial changes in the vocal cords can occur due to chronic vocal abuse coupled with irritant effects of long-term alcohol and tobacco use. The voice is described as a 'gin and midnight voice'. The changes may be reversible with vocal therapy and alteration of life habits, but most patients will require surgical removal of the hyperplastic epithelium (Fig. 3). Dysplasia or even frank neoplasia can occur in chronic hyperplastic laryngitis.

Contact ulcers

Vocal abuse due to hyperadduction of the vocal folds may result in erosion of surface mucosa; particularly susceptible is the junction of the middle and posterior third of the vocal cord (Fig. 4). These are termed contact ulcers and can be sited at the vocal process of the arytenoids. The reaction can sometimes lead to considerable granulation tissue with the formation of a contact granuloma. Gastro-oesophageal reflux may exacerbate or perpetuate this problem.

Table 1 **Non-organic causes of dysphonias**	
Type	**Cause**
Habitual dysphonias	Vocal abuse
	– acute laryngitis
	– vocal nodules
	– vocal oedema
	– chronic laryngitis
	– contact ulcer
Psychogenic dysphonias	Musculoskeletal tension disorders
	Conversion voice disorders
	– muteness
	– aphonia
	– dysphonia
	Mutational falsetto

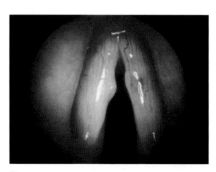
Fig. 1 **Vocal cord nodules.**

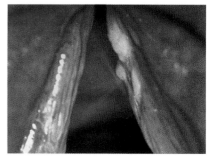
Fig. 3 **Chronic hyperplastic laryngitis due to chronic vocal abuse.** There is an area of leukoplakia on the anterior part of the right vocal cord.

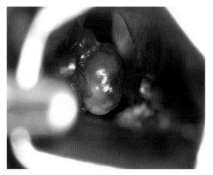

Fig. 4 **Contact ulcers are usually sited at the vocal process region of the (right) vocal cord.**

A unilateral ulcer will require biopsy to exclude neoplasia. Bilateral cases without marked granulation may resolve with vocal therapy alone. However, florid granulomas will require either surgical or laser excision with subsequent vocal training to hasten resolution and prevent recurrence.

Psychogenic dysphonia

Psychogenic dysphonias are voice disorders in the absence of laryngeal disease. The majority have an underlying anxiety or depression basis due to life stresses, personality disorders or psychoneuroses. The voice is clearly a parameter that provides clues to personality, whether normal or abnormal.

Musculoskeletal tension disorders

Tension in individuals can be due to exogenous sources, e.g. overwork, worries or family life. Endogenous causes of tension include features such as over-ambition, perfectionism and uncontrollable anger. Such stresses produce contraction of many muscle groups including the intrinsic and extrinsic muscles of the larynx. This hypertonicity results in voice disorder,

with laryngoscopic examination being normal.

The cardinal features are a dysphonia and the presence of discomfort or pain around the larynx. The clinician can reproduce the pain by palpating the larynx; quite severe pain may be elicited in this way (Fig. 5). Occasionally patients may complain of feeling a foreign body in the throat and difficulty in swallowing.

The diagnosis is confirmed by an improvement in the voice if the larynx is gently pulled down. Usually, suitable counselling to reduce the causes of stress lead to rapid resolution of symptoms. Patients in whom the voice returns to normal in certain low stress situations, e.g. on holiday, should respond rapidly to therapy.

Ventricular dysphonia (dysphonia plicae ventricularis)

Ventricular dysphonia is a voice disorder which results from utilizing the false cords to produce vibration. It is usually seen in tense individuals. However, patients with lesions of the true cords may compensate by vocalizing with the false cords. The voice is harsh and frequently low pitched as if the patient is being strangled.

Suitable speech therapy directed at muscular relaxation and correct vocalization produces good results.

Conversion voice disorders (hysterical voice disorder)

A conversion reaction is the production of physical symptoms without any underlying pathophysiological disease. If the larynx is chosen as the vehicle for the conversion reaction it can result in muteness, aphonia or dysphonia. A diagnosis of a conversion voice disorder

can only be made if the larynx is normal in structure and function. There is a background of anxiety, depression or interpersonal conflict. In the majority of cases the conversion voice disorder is associated with a major emotional conflict or stress. The voice symptoms enable the patient to avoid emotional anguish.

The basis of treatment is to uncover the causes of the stress and assist the patient in coping with the events. Retrieval of the voice must be rapid, otherwise the risk of the conversion being resistant to therapy is high.

Mutational falsetto (puberphonia)

Mutational falsetto is the failure to change from a preadolescent high-pitched voice to the lower pitched voice of male adulthood. It is rarely due to immaturity of the larynx or vocal cords. Occasionally, chronic disorders, e.g. severe childhood asthma, may prevent or retard laryngeal development. In the majority of cases of puberphonia, the larynx is anatomically and physio-logically normal.

The voice is characteristically high-pitched, weak, breathy and monotonous. There is a distinct female quality to the voice. It sounds immature and inadequately assertive. However, in sudden vocal outbursts, e.g. coughing or laughing, the voice may drop in pitch. Only a mature larynx can produce the low-pitched voice, enabling an aetiology of hypogonadism to be dismissed. Treatment produces a rapid resolution in those puberphonics who have episodes of low-pitched vocalization. In rare cases, long-term speech therapy is required to lower the fundamental speaking frequency.

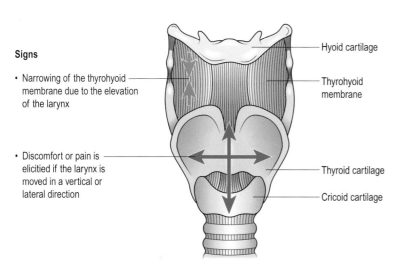

Signs

- Narrowing of the thyrohyoid membrane due to the elevation of the larynx

- Discomfort or pain is elicitied if the larynx is moved in a vertical or lateral direction

Hyoid cartilage

Thyrohyoid membrane

Thyroid cartilage

Cricoid cartilage

Fig. 5 **Laryngeal signs present in patients suffering with dysphonia secondary to musculoskeletal tension disorders.**

> ### Dysphonia – non-organic causes
>
> - Any dysphonia not resolving within 4 weeks should have a mandatory ENT referral to exclude the presence of neoplasia.
>
> - Acute onset aphonia is invariably a conversion voice disorder.
>
> - Most cases of puberphonia are psychogenic, not endocrine, in origin.
>
> - Vocal cord nodules are best treated by teaching correct vocal production. This may not be easy in young children.
>
> - Chronic non-infective laryngitis with hyperplastic epithelial changes may be a precursor of cancer. It should be biopsied.

Stridor

Definition

Stridor is noisy breathing resulting from narrowing of the airway at or below the larynx. Narrowing of the supraglottis may produce inspiratory stridor, whereas narrowing at the glottis or cervical trachea tends to produce biphasic stridor. In contrast, bronchial narrowing will produce expiratory stridor.

Stertor refers to noisy breathing due to narrowing of the airway above the larynx. An example of this is adenotonsillar hypertrophy.

Causes

Stridor results from a wide range of conditions which are summarized in Table 1 and discussed below.

General symptoms and signs of respiratory failure due to airway obstruction are given in Table 2.

Laryngotracheobronchitis

Laryngotracheobronchitis is a viral infection, usually of the parainfluenza or respiratory syncytial type, occurring mostly between ages 6 months to 3 years. Clinical features include:

- pyrexia
- a painful barking cough
- gross mucosal oedema in the lower respiratory tract
- inspiratory stridor, with two-way stridor developing in advanced stages
- complete airway obstruction in progressive cases.

The airway problems are caused by the presence of tenacious secretions and mucosal swelling in the subglottis with risk of impaction of plugs of mucus.

Hospitalization is advisable in all except the mildest cases. The child is nursed in a croupette with humidified and warmed air to loosen thick secretions. Oxygen is administered to correct hypoxia. Nebulized or systemic steroids may be helpful.

Intubation is required in progressive and severe cases. Tracheostomy is reserved for airways that cannot be intubated. Regular saline suction and physiotherapy are performed postoperatively. In most cases, endotracheal intubation should only be necessary for 2 to 5 days.

Table 1	**Age-specific causes of stridor**
Age	**Cause**
Neonatal*	Congenital tumours, cysts
	Webs
	Laryngomalacia
	Subglottic stenosis
	Vocal cord paralysis
Children*	Laryngotracheobronchitis
	Supraglottitis (epiglottitis)
	Acute laryngitis
	Foreign body
	Retropharyngeal abscess
	Respiratory papillomata
Adults	Laryngeal cancer
	Laryngeal trauma
	Acute laryngitis
	Supraglottitis (epiglottitis)

*Children are at greater risk than adults from upper airway obstruction because their airways are narrower and have softer cartilage which collapses more easily.

Table 2	**Signs of severe respiratory failure due to airway obstruction**
Cyanosis/pallor	
Nasal flaring	
Use of accessory muscles of respiration	
Tracheal plugging	
Chest wall recession	
Tachycardia	
Tachypnoea	

Supraglottitis

Supraglottitis (acute epiglottitis) is caused by Group B *Haemophilus influenzae* and is characterized by gross swelling in the supraglottis (Fig. 1). It is seen primarily in 3–7 year olds, although adults may also be affected. Clinical features include:

- pyrexia
- severe sore throat and dysphagia
- stridor
- dribbling
- breathing with raised chin and open mouth.

Supraglottitis is an emergency, as the time interval from stridor to total respiratory obstruction may be extremely short. Any distress to the child is to be avoided. Heliox and adrenaline (epinephrine) nebulizers may buy time until a senior anaesthetist and ENT surgeon are available. In most cases the anaesthetist is successful in intubating the child; however, the ENT surgeon is standing by to carry out an emergency tracheostomy if necessary. Intravenous third-generation cephalosporins are commenced and later changed depending on blood culture results. The patient is usually extubated a few days later when the condition has responded to treatment. Supraglottitis has become less common in children because of vaccination programmes.

Congenital tumours, webs and cysts

Subglottic haemangioma is the commonest congenital tumour causing stridor. It is visualized on a lateral neck X-ray. the diagnosis is confirmed by endoscopy without biopsy. The condition is self-limiting as the tumours start to regress after the first year of life, but tracheostomy is occasionally necessary for airway obstruction. Laryngeal webs or cysts of any significant size may produce stridor, particularly if the airway is further compromised by an intercurrent infection.

Laryngomalacia (congenital laryngeal stridor)

Laryngomalacia is characterized by a weak supraglottic framework which collapses on inspiration, notably during exertion and crying. Severe stridor can

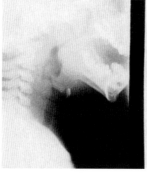
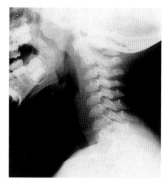

Fig. 1 **Supraglottitis.** Diagnosis is clinical and the priority is to secure the airway. Physical examination of the throat may induce respiratory arrest and should be avoided unless facilities for immediate intubation or tracheostomy are available.

Fig. 2 **Subglottic stenosis.** Seen here in a premature birth. The condition can be verified by a neck X-ray.

supervene during respiratory infections. It is self-limiting and usually resolves by the age of 2 years. Surgery may be indicated if there is failure to thrive.

Subglottic stenosis

Subglottic stenosis may be congenital. Acquired cases are the result of the trauma of prolonged endotracheal intubation, particularly in premature births (Fig. 2). Clinical features include stridor on exertion, or with respiratory infection.

Tracheostomy may be necessary to secure the airway. The subglottis can be subsequently sized and decannulation attempted if the lumen enlarges satisfactorily with age. Laser excision or laryngeal reconstructive surgery may be required in severe cases.

Foreign body obstruction

Inhalation of foreign bodies is most common in children. In adults, the problem is usually associated with psychiatric illness or alcohol intoxication. Objects can lodge anywhere in the laryngotracheobronchial tree (Fig. 3), and may remain symptomless for long periods of time. Common symptoms include:

- sudden onset of coughing, wheezing or stridor in a previously healthy child
- chest infection resulting from a foreign body in a smaller airway.

Foreign bodies can be radiolucent, so plain radiology may be misleading. Foreign bodies in the oesophagus can also produce stridor.

In a child, a foreign body may be dislodged by holding the patient up by the legs and giving a sharp slap on the back. The Heimlich manoeuvre can be used in both adults and children (Fig. 4). There should be a low threshold for tracheobronchoscopy in a child who has had a significant choking episode, even in the absence of clinical signs or radiological findings.

Retropharyngeal abscess

A now rare condition, retropharyngeal abscesses occur mostly in young infants and children. Inflammation and swelling in the retropharyngeal space, secondary to oropharyngeal infection can cause respiratory embarrassment and severe dysphagia (Fig. 5). The child assists breathing by hyperextension of the neck, which is held rigid. Urgent parenteral antibiotics are administered and surgical drainage is performed to avoid spontaneous rupture with risk of inhalation of pus.

Respiratory papillomata

Respiratory papillomata are characterized by warty lesions appearing in the larynx caused by the human papilloma virus (Fig. 6). The trachea, bronchi and pharynx may be involved in florid cases. They are thought to be due to ascending uterine infection; however, acquired cases in adults may be due to genetic predisposition or be sexually acquired. Clinical features include stridor and hoarseness.

The carbon dioxide (CO_2) laser or sharp dissection under the microscope will minimize trauma to the underlying laryngeal mucosa.

If surgery needs to be repeated frequently for symptom control, then medical therapy, such as interferons, may be considered to try to induce remission. Tracheostomy is sometimes necessary in severe cases.

Acute laryngitis

Acute laryngitis results in marked inflammation of the vocal cords which can occur in respiratory infections or secondary to vocal abuse, tobacco smoke or ingestion of spirits. Clinical features include hoarseness and throat discomfort.

Treatment is symptomatic and includes voice rest, steam inhalation and avoidance of smoke and spirits.

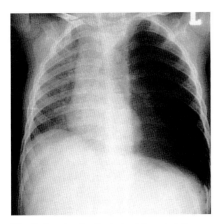

Fig. 3 **Foreign body.** A chest X-ray in full expiration. A foreign body (peanut) lodged in the left main bronchus has produced ipsilateral hyperinflation and gross mediastinal shift to the right.

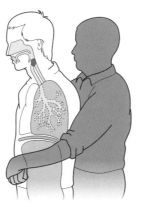

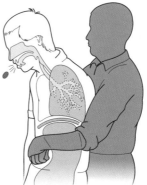

Fig. 4 **The Heimlich manoeuvre.** Performed by applying a sudden bear hug, centred on the upper abdomen and xiphisternal region.

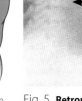

Fig. 5 **Retropharyngeal abscess.**

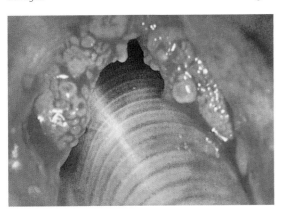

Fig. 6 **Respiratory papillomata.**

Laryngotracheal injury

The incidence of laryngotracheal trauma has decreased markedly with the compulsory wearing of car seat belts. Most injuries now occur due to sporting activities (karate, ice hockey, etc.), but also due to knives and bullets. Inhalation of smoke and ingestion of corrosive may cause severe laryngeal oedema. Clumsy laryngeal intubation for anaesthesia, or if required for long-term ventilation, may lead to chronic laryngotracheal problems (Table 1).

Injuries to the larynx are usually produced when the laryngeal framework is crushed against the bony cervical vertebrae (Fig. 1). Damage is usually more severe in the elderly where ossification reduces the resilience of the laryngeal cartilages.

Clinical features
The clinical features of laryngotracheal trauma are largely dependent on the severity of the damage. The main presenting features include:

- bleeding
- stridor
- dysphonia
- painful speech and swallowing
- surgical emphysema (Fig. 2).

Management
It is vital to consider the existence of laryngotracheal injury in trauma to the upper body. Flexible laryngoscopy is essential to provide an assessment of laryngeal damage and compromise. Maintenance and protection of the airway are major priorities in acute trauma, hence intubation or tracheostomy may be required urgently. Once the airway is secure, CT imaging should be considered to further assess the injury and early reconstruction should be planned (Table 2).

Reconstruction to preserve the laryngeal functions of airway protection and speech will require evacuation of haematomas, fixation of fractures with miniplates and sutures and stitching of mucosal surfaces.

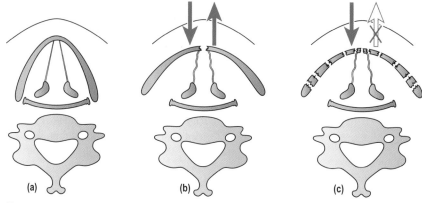

Fig. 1 **Laryngeal injury.** The type of injury depends on the type and intensity of trauma and the degree of calcification of the thyroid cartilage. **(a)** Normal laryngeal anatomy. **(b)** Uncalcified thyroid cartilage is compressed against the cervical spine. It fractures but will spring back. **(c)** A calcified thyroid cartilage shatters when compressed against the cervical spine. It does not spring back and the neck appear flattened.

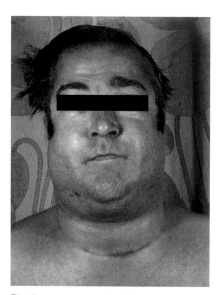

Fig. 2 **Surgical emphysema of the face, neck and upper chest in a closed injury of the larynx.**

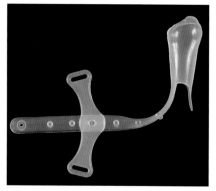

Fig. 3 **Soft Silastic stent used to support a fractured larynx** (Hood Laboratories).

Indwelling soft stents may support the laryngeal framework and prevent stenosis if left in for 1–2 weeks (Fig. 3).

Chronic laryngotracheal stenosis
In adults, chronic compromise of the airway may be due to a number of causes:

- subglottic/tracheal stenosis
- bilateral vocal cord palsies
- glottic webs.

Subglottic/tracheal stenosis
Subglottic stenosis can be congenital or acquired. The management of subglottic stenosis in children depends on the severity of the problem. Mild cases can be managed conservatively and may only require a tracheostomy until the airway has grown to an adequate size. Severe cases may require augmentation of the airway with cartilage grafts and are best managed in specialized units with a multidisciplinary approach.

Adult subglottic or tracheal stenosis is increasingly common and often

Table 1 **Causes of laryngotracheal trauma**

Type	Cause
Penetrating injuries	Knives, glass, etc.
Blunt injuries (minor & major)	Road traffic accidents Sports (karate)
Miscellaneous	Smoke inhalation Corrosive ingestion Intubation

Table 2 **Principles of treating laryngotracheal injuries**

Type of injury	Treatment
Penetrating injuries	Drain any laryngeal haematoma Exploration to remove penetrating object, e.g. bullet Reconstruct cartilage fractures
Minor blunt injuries	Observe. Intubate only if laryngeal oedema causes airway obstruction Laryngeal exploration and reconstruction may be needed
Major blunt injuries	Usually require intubation, laryngeal exploration and laryngeal reconstruction
IN ALL CASES ENSURE A SECURE AIRWAY AND CONTROL HAEMORRHAGE	

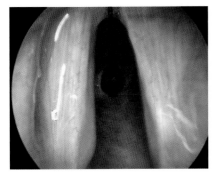

Fig. 4 **Acquired subglottic stenosis.**

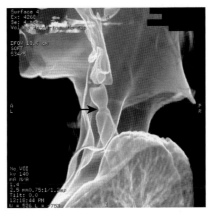

Fig. 5 **CT scan showing subglottic stenosis (arrow).**

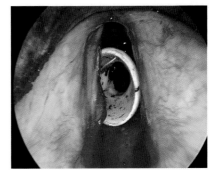

Fig. 6 **Silastic tracheal stent.**

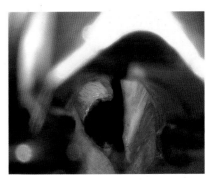

Fig. 7 **Laser cordectomy.**

misdiagnosed as asthma (Fig. 4). Advances in medical care mean that more patients are surviving periods of ventilation on intensive care units. However, injury is often sustained to the airway and one or more of the following factors may play a role:

- traumatic endotracheal intubation
- endotracheal tube too large or cuff pressures too high
- gastro-oesophageal reflux
- infection
- delay in changing to tracheostomy
- incorrectly sited tracheostomy
- some patients have an intensive inflammatory response to foreign materials in the airway.

Clinical features

These depend on the degree and site of stenosis, but include:

- dyspnoea
- stridor
- dysphonia.

Management

It is sometimes possible to visualize a subglottic stenosis using a flexible laryngoscope. The site, degree and length of the stenosis can be determined using lateral neck X-rays. A CT scan is often more helpful (Fig. 5). Respiratory function tests will help gauge the degree of disability related to the stenosis.

However, a number of patients have a tracheostomy and these tests are not always possible.

Tracheal or subglottic stenosis, if minor, may be treated with cruciate cuts using a knife or laser and dilatation. If the stenosis is more severe, it may require temporary stenting (Fig. 6).

The topical application of mitomycin C (a cytotoxic antibiotic), if used in low concentrations, can inhibit fibroblast activity and restenosis. A more severely damaged airway may require anterior augmentation or, failing this, tracheal resection and end-to-end anastomosis.

Bilateral vocal cord palsy

Bilateral vocal cord palsy may be congenital or acquired. The vocal cords come to lie in the median or paramedian position. Although voice or cry may be good, there is usually stridor and dyspnoea. Congenital bilateral cord palsy will often recover as the child grows and the only treatment necessary may be a temporary tracheostomy. Acquired bilateral cord palsy is most commonly iatrogenic, following surgery on the neck or thorax, and the patient is usually reintubated or emergency

tracheostomy carried out. It is possible to remove the tracheostomy tube following a procedure on the vocal cords. The vocal cords can either be lateralized surgically or an airway is lasered out from the back of one vocal cord (Fig. 7). The patient may subsequently be decannulated but will have a weak and 'breathy' voice.

Glottic webs

Small glottic webs can produce dysphonia and, if more severe, dyspnoea. Small webs can be managed by dividing and applying mitomycin C. The procedure may need repeating several times because the web can reform.

Larger webs are also divided but, in addition, may require the insertion of a Silastic sheet into the anterior commissure or a laryngofissure approach and the insertion of a keel (Fig. 8).

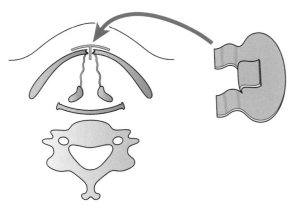

Fig. 8 **Anterior commissive injuries may lead to web formation.** A keel, made of tantalum or Silastic, can be inserted through a laryngeal fissure to prevent this complication.

Laryngotracheal injury

- Severe laryngotracheal trauma may not be associated with significant external neck signs.
- Laryngotracheal trauma may be missed if severe injury has occurred to other parts of the body.
- All laryngotracheal trauma patients should have a laryngoscopy to assess damage.
- Priority in management is protection and maintenance of the airway and arrest of haemorrhage.
- Early laryngotracheal surgery, if necessary, will largely prevent the difficult management problem of chronic laryngotracheal stenosis.

Maintenance and protection of the airway

Manoeuvres to secure the airway are required in many medical and surgical diseases. It is therefore important to be clear on the procedures available to achieve this so that potential complications may be avoided. Problems which require airway intervention include:

■ upper airway obstruction
■ protection of tracheobronchial tree
■ respiratory failure
■ elective tracheostomy in certain head and neck procedures.

Upper respiratory obstruction

Obstructive causes include:

■ infection (supraglottitis, laryngotracheobronchitis)
■ foreign bodies lodged in the larynx
■ trauma (laryngotracheal)
■ obstructing laryngeal tumours

Life-threatening respiratory obstruction

Life-threatening respiratory obstruction is usually due to inhalation of foreign bodies or infections of the laryngotrachea. Children are more likely to be involved than adults. Wide bore needles may be inserted directly into the trachea to provide temporary relief (Fig. 1) until either intubation or tracheostomy can be performed.

A similar approach is feasible with the airway entered through the cricothyroid membrane (cricothyroidotomy) (Fig. 1). The membrane is easily palpable between the cricoid ring and inferior border of the thyroid cartilage. Any sharp object, e.g. knife or scalpel, is inserted into the region and rotated once the airway is entered. Any available tube, e.g. catheter or barrel of a pen, is inserted to maintain the airway until intubation or a formal tracheostomy is performed.

It is rare nowadays to perform an emergency tracheostomy under local anaesthesia. Ongoing clinical assessment of the airway should allow it to be performed as an elective procedure.

Gradual-onset obstruction

It is imperative not to allow the clinical situation to deteriorate to one of life-threatening obstruction. Increasing stridor, the use of accessory muscles of respiration, tachypnoea, tachycardia and intercostal recession are worrying signs (Table 2 p. 65).

In all age groups endotracheal intubation should be attempted only by an experienced anaesthetist (Fig. 2). This may require additional techniques with a rigid bronchoscope or flexible laryngoscope as aids in difficult intubations. An ENT surgeon should be standing by to perform a tracheostomy if intubation fails. Tracheostomy in children should, for a variety of reasons, be avoided (Table 2, p. 70), except in an emergency.

Elective tracheostomy

The technique of elective tracheostomy is illustrated in Figure 3. The skin incision is made midway between the cricoid ring and suprasternal notch. The strap muscles are identified, running in the vertical plane, and separated in the midline. The thyroid isthmus should be divided and transfixed to avoid thyroid tissue falling into the tracheal window. In adults, a small window is then cut in the trachea between the 2nd and 3rd, or 3rd and 4th tracheal rings. In children, a vertical incision is made to avoid transecting the trachea. The cricoid cartilage and the 1st tracheal ring must not be compromised, otherwise there is a high risk of late subglottic stenosis.

An appropriate size tracheostomy tube with a high-volume low-pressure cuff should then be inserted. It is secured in position by tapes passed around the neck and tied. With the tracheostomy cuff inflated, the patient can continue to be ventilated.

Percutaneous tracheostomy tube insertion has gained popularity, especially on intensive care units. Relative contraindications to this technique include patients in whom it

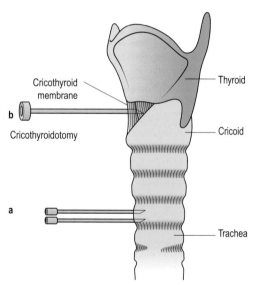

Fig. 1 **Emergency methods to secure the airway in cases of life-threatening respiratory obstruction. (a)** Needles inserted directly into the trachea. **(b)** The airway entered through the cricothyroid membrane (cricothyroidotomy; laryngotomy). In this instance a wide-bore venous cannula has been employed.

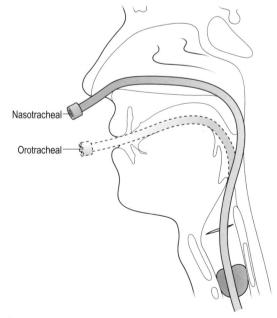

Fig. 2 **Endotracheal intubation can be routed through either the nose or the mouth.**

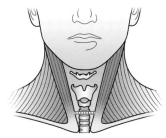

1 Horizontal skin incision midpoint between cricoid and suprasternal notch.

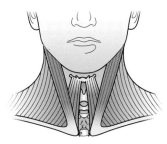

2 Strap muscles exposed and separated in midline.

Fig. 3 **Tracheostomy.**

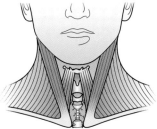

3 Strap muscles separated to expose thyroid isthmus, which is usually divided and ligated.

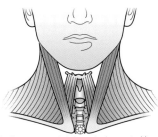

4 Trachea exposed. A fenestra is created by excising anterior tracheal rings. A simple vertical incision is used in children.

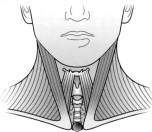

5 The opening into the trachea is ready to take the appropriate diameter tracheostomy tube.

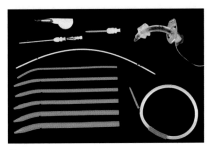

Fig. 4 **Equipment required to perform a percutaneous tracheostomy.**

is difficult to palpate the larynx and trachea (overweight) or patients with coagulopathy.

There are several percutaneous tracheostomy kits available. All are based around insertion of a needle into the cervical trachea, which allows a guide wire to be passed. An opening into the airway, large enough to insert a tracheostomy tube, is created using serial dilators (Fig. 4) or using dilation forceps or a single dilation.

The subsequent care of the tracheostomy should be meticulous in order to avoid severe complications. It is imperative to instruct the nursing staff appropriately (Fig. 1, page 70).

Protection of the tracheobronchial tree

Protection of the tracheobronchial tree, by intubation or tracheostomy, may be needed in conditions causing aspiration of pharyngeal secretions, or accumulation of bronchial secretions. This is seen in comatose states from head injury, poisoning or postneurosurgical procedures. Certain neurological conditions may weaken the ability to clear secretions, e.g. Guillain–Barré syndrome and myasthenia gravis. Aspiration of oropharyngeal secretions is seen in motor neurone disease.

After thyroid or cardio-oesophageal surgery, vocal cord paralysis can result from damage to the recurrent laryngeal nerves. If bilateral, it may cause a loss of laryngeal competence and aspiration.

Protection from bronchial secretions

With the development of medical techniques and the availability of high dependency and intensive care units, many patients are kept alive longer than previously possible. A large number of patients in such units are at risk of sputum retention, e.g. chronic bronchitics or comatose patients without a cough reflex.

The modern technique is to manage these patients by inserting a percutaneous tracheostomy (Fig. 4). This method avoids an open procedure and may be performed by either critical care clinicians or ENT surgeons.

Protection from overspill and aspiration

The most frequent causes of overspill are neoplasia of the pharyngo-oesphagus, which prevents swallowing of food and drink, and saliva. Aspiration tends to be seen in cases of uncoordinated swallowing mechanism or secondary to laryngeal incompetence. The latter may be due to either loss of vocal cord movement, usually bilateral, or reduced laryngeal sensation.

A cuffed tracheostomy tube is required to prevent oropharyngeal contents from entering the laryngotrachea. In severe cases with no prospect of recovery of laryngeal competence, a laryngectomy may be necessary.

Respiratory failure

Assisted ventilation via a secure airway will be required in cases of respiratory failure. Certain neuromuscular abnormalities preventing the mechanics of ventilation may result in respiratory failure. Damage to rib cage in severe chest injuries can also produce respiratory failure due to a 'flail chest'.

Mechanical respiratory failure may occur in isolation or together with retained bronchial secretions. If the underlying aetiology is expected to resolve within a week, endotracheal intubation is the best method to assist respiration. In all other cases, a tracheostomy will be required. This avoids complications from long-term intubation, e.g. subglottic and tracheal stenosis.

Maintenance and protection of the airway

- Life-threatening respiratory obstruction requires immediate relief. Insert needles into the trachea or perform a laryngotomy in adults.
- In children, intubate rather than perform tracheostomy.
- Sputum retention may be overcome with a 'minitracheostomy'.
- In general it is better to intubate rather than perform a tracheostomy.
- In performing a tracheostomy ensure that the cricoid cartilage and first tracheal ring are not compromised.

Postoperative care and complications of artificial airways

The old adage that 'the time to do a tracheostomy is when you first think of it' is still very apt. In acute or critical airway situations the endotracheal tube is the preferred means of securing the airway (Table 1). If it is anticipated that the patient will require ventilation for periods greater than 7–10 days, a surgical or percutaneous tracheostomy should be planned. The threshold for carrying out a tracheostomy in a child is higher than in an adult for the reasons indicated in Table 2.

Postoperative tracheostomy care

Postoperative care of a tracheostomy needs to be meticulous to avoid complications (Fig. 1). The nose assists in warming and humidifying inspired air, and this function is bypassed after tracheostomy. Copious tracheal secretions occur as a consequence and the situation is further compounded by the patient's inability to cough satisfactorily. Regular humidification prevents the formation of dried crusts. Chest physiotherapy assists in this bronchial toilet.

Crusting tends to occur at the tip and within the lumen of the tracheostomy tube. A single lumen tube requires regular removal, cleaning and reinsertion. The modern double lumen tubes have considerable

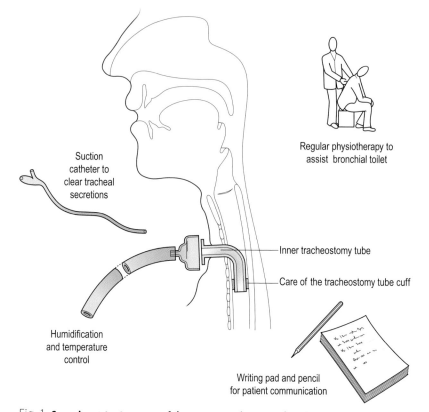

Fig. 1 **Some important aspects of the postoperative care of tracheostomy.**

(labels: Suction catheter to clear tracheal secretions; Humidification and temperature control; Regular physiotherapy to assist bronchial toilet; Inner tracheostomy tube; Care of the tracheostomy tube cuff; Writing pad and pencil for patient communication)

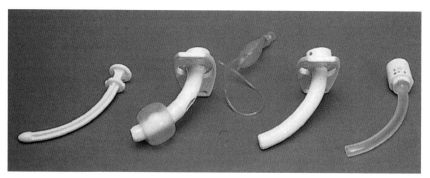

Fig. 2 **Modern tracheostomy tubes.** *From left to right:* introducer; cuffed fenestrated outer tube; uncuffed non-fenestrated outer tube; inner tube.

Table 1 **Advantages of endotracheal intubation over tracheostomy**
■ Intubation is a quicker procedure than tracheostomy
■ Clinicians skilled in intubation are more numerous and readily available than those skilled in tracheostomy
■ Tracheostomy is more easily performed in an intubated anaesthetized patient
■ The early complications of intubation are rarer and less severe than those of tracheostomy

Table 2 **Reasons for avoiding a tracheostomy in a child**
■ Most causes of respiratory obstruction in children are infective in origin and will resolve sufficiently within 72 hours to allow extubation
■ A tracheostomy is more hazardous to perform, due to a short neck, the presence of the thymus and a high brachiocephalic artery
■ Removal of a tracheostomy tube is difficult in children due to development of subglottic oedema with granulations

advantages (Fig. 2). The inner tube can be removed without disturbing the outer tube. With modern low pressure high volume cuffs, regular deflation is not required.

For the immediate postoperative period a writing pad should be provided for communication as the patient will be unable to speak. With a fenestrated tracheostomy tube a speaking valve can be fitted to help the patient talk (Fig. 3).

Complications of tracheostomy

The complications of tracheostomy are summarized in Table 3. Immediate complications include bleeding from the thyroid or anterior jugular veins. Air embolism is fortunately extremely rare.

In the postoperative period some surgical emphysema is common and is usually a result of overtight suturing of the wound. Emphysema is a problem only if it is allowed to extend from the

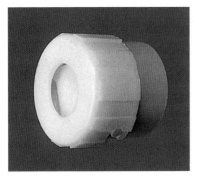

Fig. 3 **A Rusch speaking valve can be attached to the tracheostomy tube.** The valve opens in inspiration and closes in expiration so that air may flow through the glottis to allow vocalization.

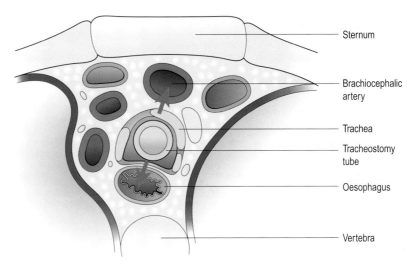

Fig. 4 **A tracheostomy tube may cause tracheal erosion anteriorly, leading to haemorrhage from the brachiocephalic artery, or posteriorly resulting in a tracheo-oesophageal fistula.**

Table 3 **Complications of tracheostomy**	
Stage	**Complication**
Operative	Haemorrhage
	Air embolism
	Cricoid injury
	Surgical emphysema
	Pneumothorax
Postoperative	
Early	Tracheitis and tracheal crusting
	Atelectasis
	Tube blockage
	Dysphagia
	Tracheal erosion
Late	Tracheomalacia
	Laryngotracheal stenosis
	Decannulation problems
	Tracheocutaneous fistula/scar

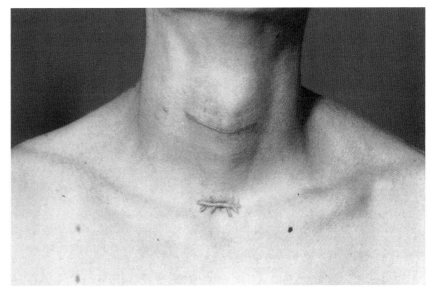

Fig. 5 **Postoperative scarring in tracheostomy.** The upper scar resulted from a laryngofissure to reconstruct the laryngeal structure after trauma. The inferior exuberant keloid scar shows the site of tracheostomy required to support the airway.

neck into the mediastinum to cause cardiopulmonary embarrassment. Mild dysphagia is common for a few days and is caused by a loss of subglottic pressure and the presence of an inflated tracheostomy cuff. If humidication is inadequate, large dried crusts may build up in the trachea and tracheostomy tube. This should be avoided by reliable humidification and regular suction clearance and physiotherapy.

Tracheal necrosis may occur due to the tracheostomy tube sitting incorrectly within the tracheal lumen. This may lead to erosion of the brachiocephalic artery and a fatal haemorrhage. Necrosis, if sited posteriorly, can result in a tracheo-oesophageal fistula (Fig. 4).

Late complications such as decannulation difficulties and tracheal stenosis may be encountered. The former is frequently due to granulations narrowing the lumen at the stomal site. Decannulation can be effected, by weaning, if the tracheal

patency is satisfactory. This involves the insertion of tracheostomy tubes of decreasing diameter until the patient can breathe with the tube occluded. Tracheal stenosis may be the end result of scarring caused by inflatable

cuffs or incorrect tracheal incisions. Skin scarring in the form of web or keloid can be unsightly. Transverse incisions made in the head neutral position result in fewer such problems (Fig. 5).

Postoperative care and complications of artificial airways

- Proper nursing care is essential after tracheostomy.
- Adequate humidification, tracheal suction as required, and physiotherapy will keep the chest free of secretions and prevent complications due to crusting.
- Most complications of tracheostomy are due to improper surgical technique, inflated cuffs or incorrectly shaped or sited tracheostomy tubes.
- All complications of tracheostomy are avoidable.

Sore throats

Sore throat is probably one of the most common symptoms encountered in medicine. Patients use the term to describe almost any feeling in the throat, ranging from dryness to actual pain. It is important therefore to ascertain the precise nature of the 'sore throat' early in the clinical history. The primary feature may be pain, but its severity may lead to dysphagia for solids, liquids and occasionally saliva. It is useful to consider separately sore throats in children and adults, although no clinical entity is exclusive to either group (Table 1).

Sore throats in adults

Acute inflammatory lesions of the pharynx are very common and settle down rapidly as the immune system, with or without antibiotics, overcomes the causative organism. Chronic sore throat in adults is much less readily understood.

Acute sore throats

Infective conditions
Viral infections of the upper respiratory tract are frequently accompanied by the same pathology affecting the pharynx. Streptococcus is occasionally the primary causative organism rather than a secondary invader following a virus. Clinically the patient complains of a painful throat. Cervical lymphadenopathy and fever are common.

If viral in origin, there is invariably a runny nose and a productive cough due to chest infection. The presence of mucopus on the pharyngeal wall implies bacterial infection. Although throat swabs are not always helpful, they may rule out bacterial infection. The treatment is symptomatic. Oral analgesics and adequate fluid intake with bed rest are required for 3–4 days to allow the disease to resolve spontaneously. Antibiotics are administered only if bacterial infection

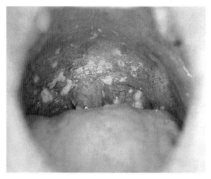

Fig. 1 **Oropharyngeal involvement with** *Candida* **in a patient with HIV infection.**

is suspected. Acute tonsillitis is uncommon in adults in comparison to its frequency in children. The clinical approach is similar in both age groups (p. 73).

Candidal infection can give rise to a painful throat and is not uncommon in the immunocomprised, e.g. diabetics, and patients undergoing radiotherapy or chemotherapy, and those afflicted by lymphomata. The acquired immune deficiency syndrome (AIDS) also increases the risk of such fungal infection. Diagnosis is made by noting typical appearance and culture (Fig. 1). Treatment may be either local antifungal agents or parenteral administration if the patient also has systemic infection.

Peritonsillar abscess
A peritonsillar abscess is a condition in which pus forms between the tonsil capsule and the superior constrictor muscle. This will be preceded by a period of peritonsillar cellulitis. The patient has symptoms of severe unilateral sore throat causing dysphagia. This may lead to inability to swallow even saliva, resulting in dribbling. The voice has a 'hot potato voice' quality. Trismus may be so prominent that visualization of the oropharynx is difficult. Ipsilateral otalgia and cervical adenopathy are other features. The most obvious clinical sign is a unilateral tonsillar inflammation causing deviation of the base of the uvula (Fig. 2).

Peritonsillar cellulitis is treated by parenteral antibiotics. If an abscess is suspected, management involves incision and drainage of the abscess and parenteral antibiotics. As the β-haemolytic streptococcus is the most frequent causative organism, penicillin is appropriate. Tonsillectomy may be advised in selected patients.

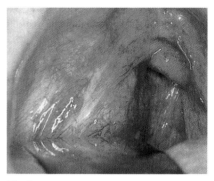

Fig. 2 **Gross swelling of the (right) tonsil due to a peritonsillar abscess.** The uvula is pushed across the midline.

Miscellaneous conditions
Blood disorders may present with lesions causing sore throats. A granulocytosis and acute leukaemia can compromise the immune system and lead to necrotic mouth and pharyngeal ulcers. The pain is usually severe and can be associated with haemorrhage. AIDS may present as recurrent acute tonsillitis or pharyngitis.

Chronic sore throats
Any patient with a chronic sore throat should be suspected of harbouring a malignancy in the oral cavity or pharynx. Associated cardinal symptoms, such as weight loss, dysphagia, hoarseness and a history of smoking and excessive alcohol intake, make such a diagnosis more likely (Fig. 1, p. 76).

The commonest cause of a chronic sore throat in adults is chronic pharyngitis. This inflammation is multifactorial and non-infective (Fig. 3). Tobacco smoke and alcohol are particularly irritant to the pharyngeal mucosa. Chronically infected tonsils, characterized by infected white debris in the tonsillar crypts, can produce a discomfort in the throat. A hiatus hernia with acid reflux can also result in a constant sore throat due to pharyngeal inflammation. Management involves conservative measures to reduce or abolish the effect of irritating agents and tonsillectomy in selected cases.

Sore throats in children

Young children are the group of patients that suffer most frequently from sore throats, and these are invariably acute in presentation.

Table 1	**Aetiology of sore throats**	
Age	**Aetiology**	
Children	Acute pharyngitis, acute tonsillitis, glandular fever, blood disorders, diphtheria	
Adults		
Acute	Tonsillitis, pharyngitis, peritonsillar abscess, candidiasis (AIDS)	
Chronic	Tonsillitis, pharyngitis (tobacco, alcohol), gastric reflux, vitamin deficiency, elongated styloid process	

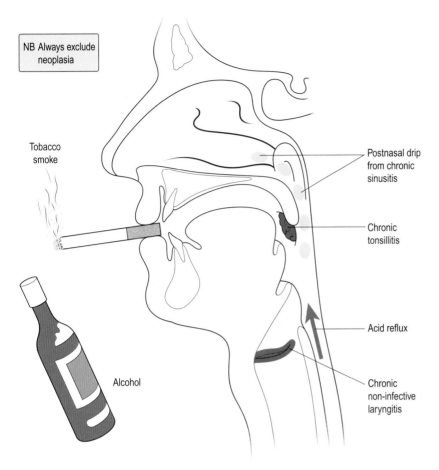

NB Always exclude neoplasia

Tobacco smoke

Postnasal drip from chronic sinusitis

Chronic tonsillitis

Acid reflux

Alcohol

Chronic non-infective laryngitis

Fig. 3 **Chronic pharyngitis: potential aetiological factors producing chronic inflammation and the symptom of sore throat.**

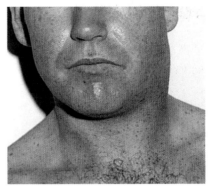

Fig. 5 **Infection of the parapharyngeal space.** This is usually due to spread from primary infection in the tonsil or teeth. There is a marked tender external swelling in the neck.

Acute sore throats

Viral infections

Viruses probably cause the majority of sore throats. A viral pharyngitis is frequently accompanied by the same organism infecting other regions of the respiratory tract, e.g. nose and trachea. The patient will thus manifest additional symptoms such as a runny nose and cough. Such cases will reveal relatively normal appearances to the tonsils. These children do not require antibiotic therapy, but are managed conservatively by ensuring sufficient fluid intake, simple analgesics and bed rest so that spontaneous resolution may occur.

Tonsillitis

Acute tonsillitis presents a quite different clinical picture. The child is systemically unwell, there is dysphagia, halitosis, pyrexia, together with cervical lymphadenopathy. The diagnosis is apparent from the appearance of the tonsils (Fig. 4). Rare disorders which give a similar appearance may need to be excluded. Diphtheria (usually the tonsil is covered by a membrane) and haematological disorders should be included in the differential diagnosis. Throat swabs are generally unhelpful

in management as the commonest organism isolated is streptococcus.

Treatment of acute tonsillitis is with bed rest and administration of antibiotics such as penicillin, with maybe the first dose parenterally. Maintenance of fluid intake is important, and paracetamol provides suitable analgesia and acts as an antipyretic in lowering the temperature. Symptoms usually resolve within a few days. Tonsillectomy may be recommended in patients with severe recurrent

infections (p. 74). Complications of tonsillitis are infrequent, but spread of infection may lead to abscess formation in peritonsillar, retropharyngeal or parapharyngeal spaces (Fig. 5).

Infectious mononucleosis

Infectious mononucleosis (glandular fever) is commonly seen in teenagers and presents as an acute sore throat. The tonsils are grossly enlarged and covered by a membranous exudate. Cervical node enlargement is gross and petechial haemorrhages may be seen on the palate. Occasionally a hepatosplenomegaly may be palpable. The diagnosis is confirmed by the presence of 'atypical lymphocytes' in peripheral blood. A positive Monospot or Paul–Bunnell test is found in the majority of cases. Treatment is symptomatic. Antibiotics are valueless, as the infective agent is the 'Epstein–Barr' virus. If ampicillin is given, due to a mistaken diagnosis of acute streptococcal tonsillitis, a skin rash develops.

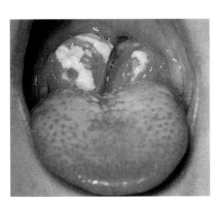

Fig. 4 **An acute bacterial tonsillitis.** Both tonsils are grossly enlarged and there is exudate on the surface. Glandular fever tonsillitis has a similar appearance.

Sore throats

- Most acute sore throats are viral in origin.
- Bacterial tonsillitis is easily diagnosed by looking at the tonsils.
- Peritonsillar abscess (quinsy) is rare in children.
- Antibiotics only shorten the course of a true bacterial tonsillitis.
- An ulcerative tonsillitis may be caused by an underlying blood disorder.
- Exclude neoplasia in any adult with a chronic sore throat.
- Think of infectious mononucleosis in teenagers, particularly if the tonsils are covered with a membranous exudate.

Tonsillectomy and adenoidal conditions

Tonsillectomy

Tonsillectomy is a very common surgical procedure in children and is frequently performed together with adenoidectomy. Tonsillectomy in adults is not infrequent.

Indications

The indications for tonsillectomy are controversial (Table 1). Recurrent tonsillitis is probably the least controversial indication, as any child having more than 3–4 attacks a year may be spending upwards of 1–2 months off school every year. Chronic tonsillitis is not a straightforward diagnosis, and some would dispute it as a cause of a chronic sore throat in adults. Tonsillectomy for peritonsillar abscess (quinsy) is only recommended if there is a past history of recurrent tonsillitis. The tonsils are usually symmetrical so that tonsillectomy for unilateral enlargement is necessary if a diagnosis of neoplasia is being entertained. More recently it has become apparent that the tonsils, usually in association with the adenoids in children and the uvulopalatal area in adults, may be a cause of snoring and the more sinister obstructive sleep apnoea. In such cases tonsillectomy may be advised, in combination with adenoidectomy and palatal surgery as appropriate (p. 80). Tonsillar biopsy is also used as a screening test for new variant Creutzfeldt–Jakob disease.

Contraindications

Contraindications to tonsillectomy are summarized in Table 1. The major operative risk is haemorrhagic so that any bleeding disorder should be corrected prior to surgery or permanent deferral may be necessary. Any recent inflammation will result in greater haemorrhage, so tonsillectomy should be avoided for 2–3 weeks after an acute infection. A child weighing less than 15 kg has a greater risk attached to the hazards of blood loss. In such cases the indications for surgery should be clear-cut and strong. Equally, a grossly overweight patient should be placed on a sensible weight reduction diet before reconsidering tonsillectomy or any other elective surgical procedure.

Procedure

The tonsillectomy is performed under general anaesthesia by dissecting the tonsil from its bed. Haemostasis is achieved using surgical ties or bipolar diathermy.

Postoperative care and complications

Postoperatively the vital signs are monitored so that any reactionary haemorrhage is quickly recognized. The patient is nursed in the tonsil or coma position until the cough reflex has recovered. Food intake is encouraged as soon as possible so that the pharyngeal muscles are prevented from stiffening, but chewing also clears slough from the tonsil beds. Post-tonsillectomy pain is still difficult to manage outside hospital and patients should be encouraged to take regular oral analgesics; local anaesthetic mouthwashes may also be helpful.

Reactionary haemorrhage occurring within the first 24 hours post-surgery is the most lethal complication. It should be picked up early provided the vital signs of blood pressure and pulse have been regularly and correctly recorded. In children the blood pressure may be well maintained due to a rise in the pulse rate until the cardiovascular system suddenly decompensates. The patient is returned to the theatre to ligate the bleeding vessel. Blood transfusion may be required.

Secondary haemorrhage is due to infective slough separating from the tonsil bed and occurs about 5–10 days post-surgery. It invariably resolves with antibiotics, only rarely requiring formal vessel ligation or transfusion.

Table 1 **Tonsillectomy: indications and contraindications**
Indications
Recurrent acute tonsillitis
Chronic tonsillitis
Peritonsillar abscess (sometimes)
Unilateral tonsillar enlargement
Snoring and obstructive sleep apnoea
Prevention of endocarditis and nephritis
Contraindications
Bleeding disorders
Recent pharyngeal infection
Weight (less than 15 kg or obesity)

The adenoids

The adenoid is a collection of lymphoid tissue in the postnasal space (Fig. 3 p. 56). Patients may attribute many symptoms to this structure, e.g. anosmia, malaise and nasal obstruction. Due to their site, adenoids in children may obstruct the Eustachian tube and may be associated with otitis media with effusion (OME). (pp. 6 and 13). Adenoidal hypertrophy is a cause of childhood nasal obstruction and discharge. The adenoid also appears to play an important role, together with the tonsils, in producing nocturnal airway narrowing which may result in obstructive sleep apnoea (p. 80).

The adenoid tends to hypertrophy up to the age of 6 years and then gradually regresses to an insignificant size by the age of about 12. Hence, pathology due to adenoidal disease is maximal by age 6 years (Fig. 1). Adults developing symptoms of adenoidal hypertrophy should have the nasopharynx examined to exclude malignancy.

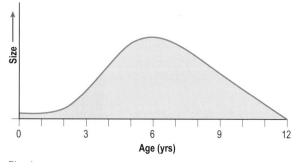

Fig. 1 **Adenoidal size in relation to age.**

Symptoms of adenoidal infection or hypertrophy
(Fig. 2)
Nasal symptoms
Large adenoids can cause severe nasal blockage resulting in mouth breathing. Other manifestations include nasal

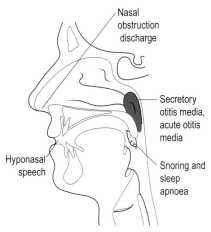

Fig. 2 **Symptoms of adenoid hypertrophy.**

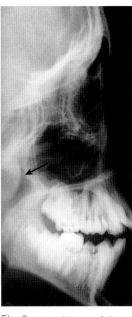

Fig. 3 **Lateral X-ray of the postnasal space showing a large pad of adenoidal tissue narrowing the airway.**

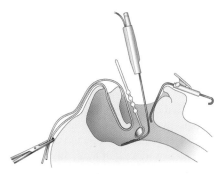

Fig. 4 **Suction diathermy and postnasal mirror used to ablate adenoidal tissue.**

discharge due to chronic adenoidal infection. Snoring and sleep apnoea in children is invariably made worse by large adenoids.

Otological symptoms

The Eustachian tube may be either physically obstructed by a large pad of adenoids or may allow an ascending infection to the ear from an adenoidal infection. The most frequent otological manifestations of such a scenario are an acute otitis media or otitis media with effusion ('glue ear').

Signs and investigations of adenoidal disease

The nasal and otological signs of adenoidal disease are fairly obvious. A child with adenoids occluding the nasopharynx may have a hyponasal voice as the nose cannot act as a resonating chamber. The child speaks as if it has a constant cold, with a low-pitched, lifeless tone.

In children a paediatric flexible nasal endoscope is the most reliable way to assess the state of the adenoids. Where this is not available, a lateral X-ray of the nasopharynx may be helpful (Fig. 3). However, in most cases a clinical assessment of relevant symptoms is sufficient to consider adenoidectomy, and the size is assessed under general anaesthesia by finger palpation of the postnasal space or a postnasal space mirror.

Adenoidectomy

The indications and contraindications to adenoidectomy are summarized in Table 2. Traditionally, adenoids are curetted under general anaesthesia, a blind technique which may leave residual adenoidal tissue. Increasingly,

adenoidectomy is performed, under vision, using a postnasal space mirror and suction diathermy ablation (Fig. 4). The postoperative care is similar to a child undergoing tonsillectomy.

Complications include reactionary haemorrhage which usually manifests as persistent nasal bleeding or occasionally haemataemesis from swallowed blood, and is accompanied by a rising pulse rate. The child is returned to theatre and a postnasal tamponade effected by a postnasal

Table 2 **Adenoidectomy: indications and contraindications**
Indications
Otitis media with effusion ('glue ear')
Chronic nasal obstruction and discharge
Sleep apnoea (with tonsillectomy)
Contraindications
Bleeding disorders
Recent pharyngeal infection
Short or abnormal palate

pack. Secondary haemorrhage is rare but occurs about 5–10 days postoperatively and usually resolves on bed rest and antibiotic therapy. Hypernasality (rhinolalia aperta) of speech can result in patients with a short palate, in whom removal of the adenoids results in air escape as the nasopharynx cannot be closed off. Such a complication is more likely in patients with a cleft palate or submucous cleft, in whom adenoidectomy should be avoided.

Tonsillectomy and adenoidal conditions

- Asymmetry in size of tonsils may be indications for tonsillectomy.
- Tonsillectomy has a mortality rate — albeit very low.
- Postoperative nursing care should be by suitably trained staff.
- Reactionary haemorrhage in the first 24 hours carries the greatest risk of morbidity and mortality.
- Tonsillectomy may fail if performed for the wrong indication, or if the tonsils are not removed in toto.
- Symptoms due to adenoidal disease are maximal at about 6 years of age.
- Secretory otitis media is frequently caused by Eustachian tube dysfunction secondary to adenoidal hypertrophy.
- Obstructive sleep apnoea and snoring in children is commonly due to both tonsils and adenoids causing airway narrowing.
- Hypernasality is a severe handicap and may result if adenoidectomy is performed in children with a short or cleft palate.
- Adenoid symptoms in adults are likely to be due to a postnasal space tumour.

Dysphagia

Dysphagia, or difficulty in swallowing, is a very common complaint. It is important to establish the precise symptoms, as a feeling of a lump in the throat is not as sinister a complaint as an actual sticking of food. Any lesion in the mouth or pharynx that disturbs the normal sequence of coordinated muscle activity or alters the anatomical structure, will cause dysphagia. Central nervous system lesions can produce dysphagia by their effect on neuromuscular activity.

Clinical features

Pharyngo-oesophageal lesions may give rise to a feeling of something in the throat, prior to the development of true dysphagia. Patients with persistence of such a sensation, particularly if associated with certain cardinal features, require full investigation (Fig. 1). Lesions in the mouth or oropharynx give a feeling of swallowing over an object, but oesophageal pathology leads to sticking of food. The duration of symptoms is important, with a progressive dysphagia being highly significant. Neurological disorders generally produce greater difficulty with swallowing liquids than solid food.

If dysphagia is present for any length of time it will lead to weight loss. Hoarseness may develop due to direct invasion of the larynx from a hypopharyngeal tumour, or subsequent to recurrent laryngeal nerve involvement. Regurgitation with dysphagia is a feature of a pharyngeal pouch. Referred otalgia is not infrequent in inflammatory and neoplastic lesions causing dysphagia.

Other features seen include aspiration with recurrent pneumonitis, particularly in pharyngo-oesophageal obstruction. Neck masses may occur due to cervical node metastases from primary malignancy in the air and food passages, or may be thyroid in origin, with secondary pharyngo-oesophageal compression causing dysphagia.

Examination

A full ENT examination is mandatory, but special attention is directed to the oral cavity, pharynx and larynx. The simple action of asking the patient to open the mouth may reveal an obvious lesion (Fig. 2). With a mirror or

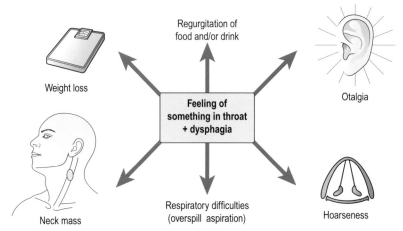

Fig. 1 **Symptoms requiring full investigation if associated with a feeling of something caught in the throat, or dysphagia.**

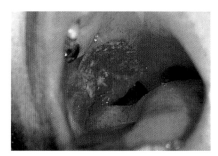

Fig. 2 **An ulcerative cancer of the right tonsil.**

flexible rhinolaryngoscope it is possible to visualize down to the laryngopharynx, which may show pooling saliva or a vocal cord paralysis. Careful palpation of any local lesion and the neck is essential.

Investigations

The principal investigation is a barium swallow which outlines the hypopharynx, oesophagus and stomach (Fig. 3). A plain lateral X-ray of the neck may reveal shadowing due to neoplasia of the posterior pharyngeal wall. In persistent dysphagia, even with normal radiological tests, a pharyngo-oesophagoscopy is mandatory. Any abnormal lesion must be biopsied.

Acute dysphagia

Acute dysphagia is very common and can be due to inflammatory conditions such as tonsillitis (p. 72) or aphthous ulceration (p. 82). Other causes include swallowed foreign bodies or the ingestion of caustic liquids. A diagnosis of the aetiology is made relatively easily from the history.

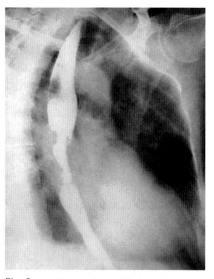

Fig. 3 **A mid-oesophageal lesion showing a filling defect on a barium swallow.**

Chronic dysphagia

Patients with chronic dysphagia require an in-depth history and examination as already discussed. The causes of chronic dysphagia are listed in Table 1.

Neuromuscular disorders

Dysphagia is invariably associated with other manifestations of the underlying pathology. Neurological lesions frequently cause sensory denervation of the larynx with a high risk of aspiration. Motor neurone disease results in a similar risk to the airway because of severe incoordination of the swallowing mechanism. Division of the cricopharyngeus (cricopharyngeal myotomy) may relieve dysphagia of neurological origin, as there is a failure

Table 1	**Causes of chronic dysphagia**
Type	**Cause**
Neuromuscular disorders	Motor neurone disease, multiple sclerosis, myasthenia gravis
Intrinsic lesions	Neoplasia, pharyngeal pouch, strictures, achalasia
Extrinsic lesion	Thyroid enlargement, aortic aneurysm
Systemic causes	Scleroderma (rare)
Psychosomatic	Globus pharyngeus

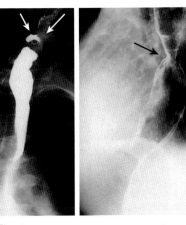

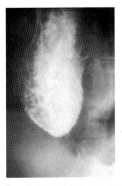

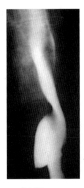

Fig. 4 (left) **A small pharyngeal pouch (arrows) that retains contrast medium during a barium swallow.**

Fig. 5 (right) **A stricture of the lower third of the oesophagus due to long-standing oesophageal reflux.**

Fig. 6 (left) **Achalasia of the cardia.** The oesophagus is grossly dilated containing food and liquid debris. The distal part of the oesophagus is extremely narrow.

Fig. 7 (right) **Dysphagia lusoria.** This very rare cause of dysphagia is due to an aberrant right subclavian artery coursing posterior to the oesophagus, causing a spiral filling defect.

of this segment of the lower pharynx to relax.

Intrinsic lesions of the digestive tract

Neoplasia
Neoplasia of the pharyngo-oesophagus is a frequent cause of dysphagia and is invariably associated with other cardinal features (Fig. 1; see also p. 106). The common sites affected are the piriform fossa, postcricoid region and the oesophagus. The majority of cases will require radiotherapy and salvage surgery. The resected portion of the pharyngo-oesophagus can be replaced by either a portion of jejunum or the stomach pulled into the defect and anastomosed to the superior resection margin. In some cases the larynx is also removed so that the patient breathes through the trachea which is relocated to the anterior neck.

Pharyngeal pouch
A pharyngeal pouch is a hernia of the pharyngeal mucosa through a potential weakness (Killian's dehiscence) between the upper thyropharyngeus and lower cricopharyngeus fibres of the inferior constrictor muscle. Food debris collects in the pouch, which enlarges progressively. Regurgitation of undigested food particles is common and overspill may result in a chronic cough and pneumonitis. The pouch may increase in size to such an extent that it compresses the oesophagus to cause dysphagia. A barium swallow is usually diagnostic (Fig. 4). All but the smallest pouches will require either surgical excision and cricopharyngeal myotomy through the neck, or endoscopic stapling and division of the party wall between the pharynx and oesophagus.

Oesophageal stricture
Strictures of the oesophagus may be due to malignancy or secondary to fibrosis induced by chronic reflux oesophagitis associated with a hiatus hernia. It is important to fully investigate all strictures with biopsy, to exclude neoplasia. Inflammatory strictures

producing dysphagia are invariably accompanied by a long history of heartburn and epigastric discomfort. The typical stricture due to oesophageal reflux is seen in the lower third of the oesophagus (Fig. 5). Treatment comprises aggressive medical therapy to counteract the acid reflux, and possible dilatation of the stricture. Failure of conservative measures in patients with severe symptoms will necessitate surgical correction.

Achalasia of the oesophagus
Achalasia of the oesophagus is caused by a failure of relaxation of the cardia and abnormal oesophageal muscular tone during swallowing. This results in a stricture at the defective site, with gross proximal dilatation of the oesophagus. Besides dysphagia, regurgitation is common. A barium swallow has a typical appearance (Fig. 6). The majority of patients will require a cardiomyotomy (Heller's operation) to divide the cardiac sphincter, as dilatation with bougies frequently fails to produce satisfactory relief.

Extrinsic lesions
The thyroid gland may narrow the oesophagus, either by compression in benign pathology, or by direct invasion in cases of malignancy. Vascular compression of the oesophagus can be produced by an aortic aneurysm or an aberrant right subclavian artery (dysphagia lusoria) (Fig. 7).

Psychosomatic causes
Globus pharyngeus, previously called globus hystericus, is a condition mainly of middle-aged women who complain

of a feeling of lump in the throat. True dysphagia is not present. the patient usually volunteers that the symptoms are noted particularly during periods of anxiety. In such cases reassurance is all that is required. However, in those patients that appear to be psychologically well-balanced, a barium swallow and a diagnostic oesophagoscopy should be performed to exclude neoplasia. It is now felt that in many cases of globus pharyngeus, acid reflux produces a reflex cricopharyngeal spasm leading to the symptom complex. It is therefore reasonable to give a trial of antireflux treatment, which may include simple antacids and proton pump inhibitors.

Dysphagia

- A persistent feeling of something in the throat requires full investigation.

- Insist on establishing beyond doubt that a patient has true dysphagia.

- Always ask about the cardinal associated symptoms.

- Acute dysphagia is usually inflammatory in origin, but exclude a foreign body, particularly in children.

- All cases of chronic dysphagia require endoscopy, even in the presence of a normal barium swallow.

- Neurological causes of dysphagia are notoriously difficult to manage.

- Ensure that benign oesophageal strictures are truly benign by biopsy.

- Many persistent cases of globus pharyngeus will require barium swallow and endoscopy.

- A trial of therapy to neutralize or decrease gastric secretions may benefit patients with a globus pharyngeus.

Salivary glands

Pathology of the major salivary glands, the parotids and submandibular glands, will present usually as a swelling which may be associated with pain. It is important to establish the characteristics of any swelling, particularly to note if it is intermittent, constant or progressive. Most causes of salivary disease producing pain are exacerbated by chewing. The major salivary glands are anatomically closely associated with lymph nodes, so non-salivary gland pathology may mimic salivary gland disease. It is important to appreciate that enlargement of the deep lobe of the parotid gland may cause swelling in the tonsil region which may not be visible or palpable in the neck (Fig. 1).

Minor salivary glands are located in the oral cavity and palate. In the mouth they frequently cause salivary retention cysts. (p. 83).

Parotid gland

Swelling
The parotid gland territory is more extensive than most clinicians appreciate. Parotomegaly can affect the gland diffusely, or be localized to one area (Table 1). Extraparotid disease

Table 1 Causes of swelling and pain of the parotid gland	
Symptom	**Cause**
Swelling	Extraparotid (Fig. 1)
	Parotid
	■ neoplasia
	■ Sjögren's
	■ sarcoidosis
	■ systemic diseases
	■ drugs
Swelling and pain	Mumps parotitis
	Bacterial parotitis
	Sialectasis
	Neoplasia
	Calculus

may present as parotid lumps (Fig. 1). A unilateral localized swelling is invariably neoplastic, of which 90% will be benign pleomorphic adenomas. Malignant parotid tumours are frequently accompanied by pain and facial nerve paresis, in addition to parotomegaly (see p. 113).

Sjögren's syndrome
Bilateral parotid swelling with little or no pain is a feature of Sjögren's syndrome. It is associated with xerostomia (dry mouth), keratoconjunctivities sicca (dry eyes) and rheumatoid arthritis. Other salivary glands may be similarly affected. It

appears to be an autoimmune disease. The diagnosis is made by showing typical histological appearance on sublabial biopsy of minor salivary glands. Treatment is symptomatic, e.g. instillation of artificial tears and saliva. Patients with Sjögren's syndrome run an increased risk of developing a parotid lymphoma.

Sarcoidosis
Sarcoidosis is a multisystem disease and may affect the parotid gland. The swelling is diffuse and is frequently associated with uveitis. The diagnosis is made either by biopsy of the gland, or more readily by seeing specific histological changes in the nasal turbinates. Serum angiotensin-converting enzyme levels are raised in sarcoidosis.

Other causes of parotomegaly
A variety of systemic diseases and drugs may be associated with parotomegaly (Table 2).

Swelling and pain
Most patients who complain of pain in the parotid region invariably exhibit some degree of swelling. Most causes of parotid pain are exacerbated by chewing and this can be elicited by requesting the patient to chew a lemon flavoured sweet.

Mumps
This used to be the most common cause of bilateral parotid swelling until the introduction of vaccination programmes (Fig. 2). Mumps-related parotomegaly is tender to touch and there is usually trismus and pyrexia. Treatment is symptomatic unless a bacterial infection supervenes to produce suppuration. Rare complications of mumps infection

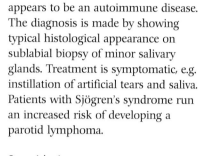

Masseter
Mandible
Parotid gland
Facial nerve
External carotid artery
Carotid canal
Mastoid process

Tonsil
Oral cavity
Cervical vertebra

① Winged mandible
② Masseteric hypertrophy
③ Lipoma
④ External carotid aneurysm

Fig. 1 **Extraparotid causes of parotomegaly.**

Table 2 Systemic and drug causes of parotomegaly	
Type	**Cause**
Systemic disease	Obesity
	Hypothyroidism
	Cushing's syndrome
	Gout
	Diabetes mellitus
Drugs	Oestrogen contraceptive pill
	Dextropropoxyphene
	Alcohol

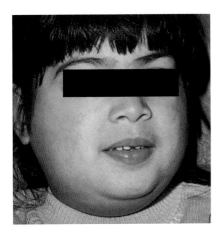

Fig. 2 **Bilateral parotid enlargement due to mumps virus infection.**

include orchitis and sensorineural deafness.

Bacterial infection

A bacterial parotid infection is usually unilateral. The victim is commonly elderly and debilitated, or may be recuperating after surgery. The whole gland is enlarged, exquisitely tender and pus may be seen in the parotid duct orifice intraorally. Treatment consists of high-dose parenteral antibiotics, and surgical drainage if pus is present.

Neoplasia

Neoplasia, particularly if malignant, presents with parotid pain and swelling (p. 112). Secondary bacterial infection may produce features of a parotitis. The facial nerve is commonly affected, and there may be skin tethering (Fig. 3).

Sialectasis

Sialectasis, causing destruction and loss of the parotid duct system, is a common cause of recurrent bouts of pain and swelling. Many patients have minimal symptoms that do not require treatment. Parotidectomy is indicated in patients with significant symptoms, particularly if associated with calculi.

Parotid calculi

Calculi of the parotid gland are much rarer than in the submandibular gland. Surgical intervention may be necessary.

Submandibular gland

Swelling

Painless diffuse enlargement of the submandibular gland is infrequent. In such cases, neoplasia should be excluded (Table 3).

Swelling and pain

The commonest cause of swelling in the submandibular gland region is secondary to infection in the oral cavity. This is because the gland is associated with lymph nodes which become involved in the inflammatory response. Apical infection of the lower

molars, gum disease and metastatic intraoral cancer may all produce swelling in this area.

Submandibular calculi

The commonest primary disease of the submandibular gland causing pain and swelling is calculi. The symptoms are typically related to meal times. Usually the distal part of the duct is blocked so that many calculi are palpable in the floor of the mouth. Most stones are radio-opaque (Fig. 4). If located in the mouth they can be removed by an intraoral approach. More proximally sited calculi require excision of the gland.

Neoplasia

Any localized swelling of the submandibular gland, especially if painful, is almost certainly of malignant aetiology. Benign tumours of this gland are much less frequent than in the parotid.

Table 3 **Causes of swelling and pain of the submandibular gland**

Symptoms	Cause
Swelling	Neoplasia
Swelling and pain	Intraoral disease causing lymph node involvement (giving rise to these symptoms in the submandibular region)
	Calculus
	Neoplasia

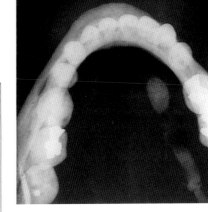

Fig. 4 **A stone in the submandibular duct.**

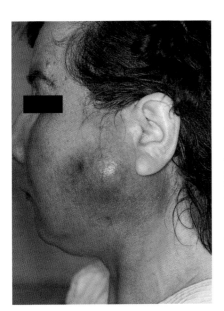

Fig. 3 **Adenocarcinoma of the parotid gland.**

Salivary glands

- One of the commonest causes of bilateral parotid swelling is mumps parotitis.
- An acute unilateral diffuse swelling of the parotid is nearly always a bacterial parotitis.
- Localized parotid swellings may be neoplastic.
- The majority of neoplastic parotid swellings are benign.
- Progressive pain, skin tethering and facial nerve involvement are indicative of a malignant parotid lesion.
- The commonest cause of swelling and pain in the region of the submandibular gland is intraoral disease.
- Submandibular calculi are the commonest cause of recurrent pain and swelling of the submandibular gland.
- Localized swellings of the submandibular gland, with or without pain, should be assumed to be malignant until proven to the contrary.

Snoring and sleep apnoea

Introduction

Sleep-related breathing disorders are now more readily identified due to the establishment of sleep laboratories and a general awareness of sleep-related pathology. Such disorders may produce subtle changes with potentially lethal long-term consequences. Snoring in particular was regarded as a rather comical nocturnal manifestation, but it is now appreciated that it may precipitate more profound cardiorespiratory problems.

Snoring may be produced by vibration of pharyngeal structures such as tongue, soft palate and pharyngeal walls. In adults, *sleep apnoea* is defined as 30 episodes of cessation of breathing for a duration of at least 10 seconds over a 7-hour period of sleep. The condition is less well defined in children and shorter periods of apnoea may be significant.

Sleep apnoea may be secondary to three situations:

- *Central sleep apnoea*, the most uncommon, is due to a defect in the respiratory drive centre in the brain stem.
- *Obstructive sleep apnoea (OSA)* frequently presents to the ENT department, either labelled as snoring or sometimes snoring with apnoea. In OSA, unlike central sleep apnoea, there are chest movements and a struggle to shift air, but without success. The site of the airway obstruction in OSA may be nasal, pharyngeal or laryngotracheal (Fig. 1).
- *Mixed-type sleep apnoea* has manifestations of both the central and obstructive types.

The relevance of snoring is that it may be a precursor to obstructive sleep apnoea. Some patients may be tipped into a full-blown sleep apnoeic state if sedated, e.g. by ingestion of alcohol or sedative drugs.

Potential complications

Potential complications of obstructive sleep apnoea are summarized in Table 1. A partial airway obstruction, producing snoring or a full-blown apnoeic episode, causes oxygen desaturation. If this continues long term, it may result in a pulmonary hypertension, eventually leading to right ventricular failure and cor pulmonale.

The disruption of normal sleep patterns produces a state of sleep deprivation in the patient. This can result in daytime lethargy, hypersomnolence and loss of memory and concentration. Children with obstructive sleep apnoea may also display failure to thrive. Obstructive events lead to multiple arousals from sleep. The growth hormone surge occurs during the later stages of sleep and these children may not spend sufficient time in deep sleep. There may also be a link between sleep apnoea and sudden infant death syndrome (SIDS).

Table 1 **The potential complications of obstructive sleep apnoea**	
Type	**Complication**
Cardiac	Raised pulmonary artery pressure
	Pulmonary hypertension
	Cor pulmonale
	Cardiac dysrhythmias
CNS	Hypersomnolence
	Lethargy
	Reduced concentration and memory
General	Sudden infant death syndrome (cot death)
	Failure to thrive (children)

Clinical signs

Obstructive sleep apnoea (OSA)

Snoring is invariably present. It is usually loud but interspersed with the apnoeic episodes when the pharynx is totally occluded. There is a struggle, with limbs thrashing in an attempt to shift air, and considerable movement of the thorax and abdomen is apparent. Symptoms due to sleep deprivation and secondary cardiac complications may occur.

The adult patient is frequently overweight and has a short neck, but routine examination may be normal. In children the tonsils may be so large that they meet or 'kiss' in the mid-line.

Central sleep apnoea

In contrast to OSA, there is no struggle in these patients. However, the features of sleep deprivation and any associated CNS pathology may be present.

Sites of obstruction		Causes of obstruction
Nose/naso-pharynx		Nasal polyps
		Grossly deflected nasal septum
		Adenoids
Oropharynx/velopharynx		Macroglossia (absolute or relative)
		Soft palate
		Tonsils
Laryngotrachea		Obstructive lesions (e.g.tumour, cysts)

Fig. 1 **Potential sites and causes of narrowing that may result in snoring and obstructive sleep apnoea.**

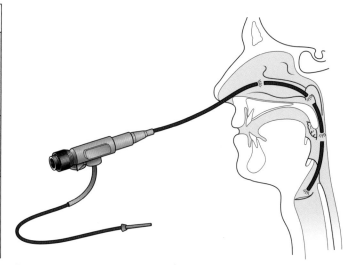

Fig. 2 **Examination with the flexible rhinolaryngoscope.** A full examination of the upper respiratory tract may allow identification of the obstructive causes of snoring and sleep apnoea.

Investigations

A full ENT investigation is mandatory to discover any cause of obstruction of the upper respiratory tract and should include sleep nasendoscopy. The patient with central sleep apnoea should be referred for a neurological opinion and management.

Rhinolaryngoscopy

Passage of a flexible rhinolaryngoscope (Fig. 2) allows a full examination of the upper respiratory tract to identify any obstructive pathology. It can also be employed to observe if the velopharyngeal lumen is compromised as a patient recovers from a short anaesthetic which mimics sleep nasendoscopy. A forced negative Valsalva (Müeller manoeuvre) with visualization of the velopharynx also provides a measure of potential narrowing in this region.

Radiology and CT scanning

Radiological investigation may be a simple lateral X-ray of the postnasal space to identify an adenoidal pad, and other views to check the position and size of the tongue in relation to the jaw. CT scanning can also be used to assess airway obstruction.

Sleep studies

The routine investigations may be inconclusive, and a satisfactory screening evaluation should include a sleep study.

During the sleep study it is possible to measure the following parameters (Fig. 3):

- cutaneous oxygen saturation levels to detect any hypoxic dips
- ECG monitors to assess the presence of arrhythmias and other cardiac abnormalities during periods of hypoxia
- air movement with nasal thermistors or by direct observation
- chest wall and abdominal movements detected by strain gauges.

Management of obstructive sleep apnoea

Medical treatment may be given a trial in patients with mild snoring and sleep apnoea. A reduction in weight and alcohol intake may produce some benefit. Medications include respiratory stimulants or those designed to reduce the period of REM sleep during which the patient is at greatest risk of developing apnoea. However, severe symptoms require more urgent treatment. Continuous positive airway pressure (CPAP) may be used to prevent pharyngeal collapse. It involves blowing air into the respiratory tract via the nose and aims to reduce apnoeic episodes and prevent significant oxygen desaturation. The improvement can be dramatic but it may be poorly tolerated by patients. Palatal and tonsillar surgery or mandibular advancement splints may have a role in mild obstructive sleep apnoea.

Surgery

In adults, nasal surgery may be required for nasal polyposis or a deflected septum. The velopharyngeal isthmus is also frequently the site of narrowing, and this is corrected by either a laser-assisted palatoplasty (LAPP) or a uvulopharyngopalatoplasty (UPPP) with a tonsillectomy (Fig. 4). The results of these procedures on snoring and sleep apnoea are variable. Some patients may be candidates for hyoid and jaw surgery to correct obstruction at other levels.

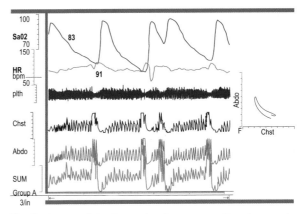

Fig. 3 **Sleep study in obstructive sleep apnoea.** Note the apnoeic episodes associated with severe hypoxaemia (SaO$_2$), and the elevated heart rate (HR). The chest and abdominal wall distortion increases with developing desaturation.

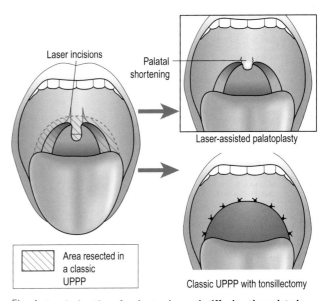

Fig. 4 **Surgical options for shortening and stiffening the palate in snoring and upper airway obstruction.**

In extreme cases of OSA, a tracheostomy may be life-saving, as it provides a bypass to any obstruction.

In children the usual site of narrowing is the oropharynx caused by hypertrophy of the tonsils and adenoids. This is easily corrected by adenotonsillectomy. Sedatives premedication must be avoided.

Snoring and sleep apnoea

- Snoring may not be a trivial noise.
- Sleep apnoea may be central, obstructive or mixed.
- OSA is always associated with snoring.
- Patients with OSA manifest a struggle during episodes of apnoea.
- Persistent sleep apnoea may result in serious cardiac and central nervous system complications.
- A sleep study is a useful screening procedure, both in snorers and patients with suspected sleep apnoea.
- Adenotonsillectomy is all that is required to cure the majority of children with OSA.
- A tracheostomy may be life-saving in severe OSA.

Oral cavity

The symptoms and signs of oral disease have already been covered (p. 58). Most lesions will either be visible to both patient and clinician, or easily palpable. The commonest intraoral pathologies are dental caries and periodontal disease.

Congenital and developmental anomalies

Congenital and developmental anomalies are not uncommon in the oral cavity. Abnormal development of the frenulum may result in tongue-tie (*ankyloglossia*). If it interferes with articulation, which is extremely rare, it can be freed surgically. *Macroglossia* is usually seen in association with mongolism. However, it is also a feature of acromegaly. Vascular and lymph vessel abnormalities can result in macroglossia (Fig. 1).

Cleft palate

The commonest development defects of the palate are clefts. These may be complete and involve the lips, alveolus and palate. The repair of the cleft lip is performed as soon as possible after birth. The palatal defect is closed at about 6–12 months. The repair will also involve lengthening the soft palate so that the nasopharynx can be closed from the oropharynx to prevent nasal escape of air during speech, and nasal regurgitation of food and liquids during eating.

Ulceration in the oral cavity

Recurrent oral ulceration

Recurrent ulceration is the commonest cause of ulcers in the oral cavity. It may be due to aphthous ulceration which is of unknown aetiology, although nutritional and hormonal factors, as well as minor trauma, have been implicated. Herpes simplex eruptions have similar clinical features, although are more likely to involve the hard palate. Some patients with recurrent oral ulceration may have underlying vitamin B, folic acid or iron deficiencies. The lesions usually commence as a small vesicle which rapidly progresses to form ulcers. They may be of any size and number and occur anywhere in the mouth (Fig. 2). There is severe pain and the ulcers resolve spontaneously after 2–3 weeks. Various steroid preparations as pastes or pellets may be used orally to treat ulcers. Mouthwashes containing

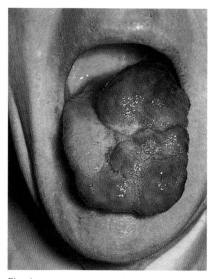

Fig. 1 **A congenital cavernous haemangioma causing gross macroglossia.**

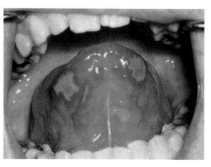

Fig. 2 **Aphthous ulceration of the tongue.**

antibiotics or antiseptics give some pain relief, e.g. phenol gargles. Treatment with aciclovir may be employed in ulcers of herpetic origin.

Infectious ulceration

Specific microorganisms may cause oral ulceration. Tuberculosis in the oral cavity is now rare. Syphilitic disease has oral manifestations. The primary chancre has a typical appearance. Snail track ulcers may occur in the secondary stage and gummatous eruptions of the tertiary stage may affect the palate.

Acute ulcerative stomatitis (Vincent's angina) is an infection with a spirochaete and an anaerobic organism. It is seen in patients with poor nutrition, low general resistance and inadequate oral hygiene. The ulceration occurs along the gingival margins but spreads and coalesces. There is a marked foetor. Treatment involves penicillin and metronidazole given intravenously, and attention to oral hygiene and nutrition.

Other causes of ulceration

Potential neoplastic causes of oral ulceration should never be overlooked, particularly if the ulcer persists, enlarges or is associated with cervical adenopathy.

Certain haematological diseases may cause intraoral ulceration. Agranulocytosis can present with an acute sore throat or tongue ulceration, and acute lymphatic leukaemia may be associated with haemorrhage and ulceration of the gum margins.

Autoimmune diseases can give rise to oral manifestations. Reiter's syndrome produces arthritis, ocular lesions and oral ulceration. Behçet's syndrome consists of orogenital ulceration and uveitis. The oral lesions in both conditions are treated with steroid preparations to reduce the inflammation and provide pain relief.

White lesions in the oral cavity

The three commonest white lesions in the mouth are:

- lichen planus
- candidiasis
- leukoplakia.

Lichen planus may be clinically and histologically difficult to distinguish from leukoplakia (Fig. 3). Both can occur anywhere in the oral cavity, although lichen planus may be associated with a variable degree of pain. Biopsy is essential to differentiate the two lesions and also to exclude the presence of malignancy in cases of leukoplakia. Between 3 and 5% of leukoplakic plaques are premalignant and this is more likely in females who smoke.

Candidiasis occurs in the very young, debilitated adults, patients on broad-spectrum antibiotics, and those

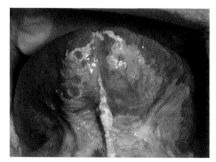

Fig. 3 **Extensive white patches on the tongue mucosa.** This is due to leukoplakia, but lichen planus may have an identical appearance.

who are immunocompromised. The typical lesions are white plaques which tend to coalesce into a membrane. If the membrane is removed a raw bleeding area is left. Local treatment with fungicides in tablet or solution form produces rapid resolution.

White leukoplakic patches, usually localized to the lateral border of the tongue, are frequently seen in AIDS (acquired immune deficiency syndrome). Due to the histological features, such lesions are termed 'hairy leukoplakia'. They are caused by an Epstein–Barr virus infection.

Red lesions in the oral cavity
Geographical tongue
Geographical tongue (erythema migrans linguae) has a typical appearance. There are numerous red patches which gradually coalesce, but characteristically the patterns change with time. In the red areas there is an absence of filiform papillae. The condition is asymptomatic and usually remits spontaneously.

Median rhomboid glossitis
Median rhomboid glossitis appears as a smooth red patch over the mid-dorsum of the tongue. The area lacks papillae or taste buds and is sometimes associated with candidiasis.

Vitamin deficiencies
Deficiencies of vitamin B (riboflavin and nicotinic acid) produce pellagra. This results in smooth red lips (cheilitis) and a painful glossitis. Vitamin C deficiency gives rise to scarring which is associated with severe swelling and bleeding of the gums.

Scarlet fever
Scarlet fever may present in association with acute streptococcal tonsillitis. However, it may be accompanied by the 'strawberry tongue' with or without the skin rash.

Cystic lesions in the oral cavity
Retention cysts
Retention cysts can occur due to duct blockage of a minor salivary gland. They can reach considerable sizes, particularly if located in the floor of the mouth, when the term 'ranula' is applied (Fig. 4). A localized lymphangioma has an identical appearance.

Fordyce spots
Fordyce spots can occur in upwards of 50% of the population by adult life.

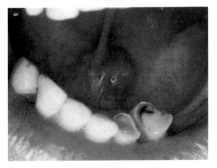

Fig. 4 **A mucous retention cyst (ranula) in the floor of the mouth.**

They are small yellow spots, usually in the buccal mucosa, and are caused by heterotopic sebaceous glands.

Pemphigoid eruptions
Pemphigus and mucous membrane pemphigoid both cause transitory cystic lesions, but they are more likely to present as relapsing oral ulceration. The diagnosis is made by biopsy of the para-ulcer tissue. Treatment involves systemic steroids.

Torus palatinus
A bony exostosis of the posterior portion of the hard palate, a torus palatinus (p. 58), may alarm a patient. They are benign and can be removed if affecting dentures.

Miscellaneous lesions in the oral cavity
Radiotherapy
A potent cause of intraoral problems is external beam radiotherapy. It can lead to a dried, inflamed and cracked oral mucosa, covered in thick tenacious secretion. The tongue can take on a smooth appearance due to papillae loss.

Fissured tongue
A fissured tongue is frequently a congenital condition (Fig. 5). On rare occasions it is associated with iron deficiency anaemia. Most cases are asymptomatic, but if food debris collects in the grooves it may give rise to soreness and halitosis. This is easily managed by regular oral hygiene.

Black hairy tongue
A black hairy tongue is caused by an overgrowth of filiform papillae on the dorsum (Fig. 6). Most sufferers are tobacco smokers and some cases have followed local application of antibiotics. The papillae may reach 1 cm in length and are treated by scraping and daily application of a toothbrush to the tongue.

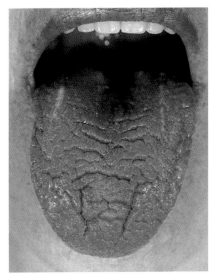

Fig. 5 **Fissured tongue.**

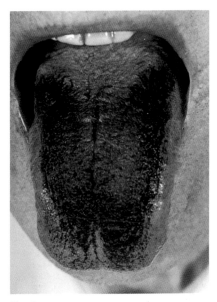

Fig. 6 **A severe case of black hairy tongue.**

Intraoral lumps
Although most lumps in the oral cavity are diagnosed clinically, neoplasia may present as a mass rather than an ulcer. This is especially true of tongue lumps. Therefore, virtually all intraoral lumps should be biopsied.

> ## Oral cavity
> - All lesions in the oral cavity, visible or not, should be palpated.
> - Lesions in the mouth may be due to local or systemic disease.
> - Lichen planus and leukoplakia may look indentical.
> - Leukoplakia may be premalignant and therefore should be biopsied.
> - All persistent ulcers and any non-ulcerating masses should be biopsied to exclude neoplasia.

Foreign bodies

Foreign bodies may be inhaled or swallowed. Inhaled foreign bodies are most frequently seen in young children. Swallowed objects are also seen in the younger age group, but may be encountered in the elderly and psychiatrically disturbed.

Inhaled foreign bodies

Over 75% of patients presenting with inhaled foreign bodies are children aged 4 years or under. The features of foreign body inhalation are dependent on its type and location in the laryngotracheobronchial tree. Vegetable material, e.g. peanuts, seeds and popcorn, produce a severe mucosal reaction in comparison to inorganic material, e.g. coins and buttons. Impaction in the larynx may be rapidly fatal due to complete respiratory obstruction. The Heimlich manoeuvre may dislodge the object and should be attempted. In other circumstances an alternative airway should be secured (p. 66), and the foreign body removed endoscopically.

Clinical features

There is initially an episode of choking and coughing which is associated with wheezing. Tracheal location of the object will produce bilateral wheezing, but bronchial sites give unilateral symptoms. Thereafter the patient may remain asymptomatic for days, weeks or months. Symptoms manifest only as a consequence of the mucosal reaction producing obstruction. Vegetable foreign bodies generally present earlier because of this physiological response.

The diagnosis of an inhaled foreign body should always be considered in a child who, being previously healthy, develops sudden-onset wheezing. The history is usually suggestive.

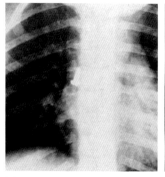 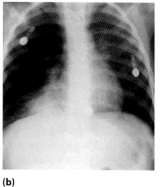

(a)   **(b)**

Fig. 1 **Inhaled foreign bodies. (a)** A radio-opaque foreign body (metal screw) located in the right bronchial tree. **(b)** An inhaled body in the right lower respiratory tract causing hyperventilation of the ipsilateral lung with loss of lung markings.

Signs such as unilateral wheezing, poor chest movement and reduced breath sounds may be elicited.

It is essential to perform a chest X-ray in expiration. This investigation may show signs of hyperinflation, infection and collapse. The foreign body may or may not be radio-opaque (Fig. 1).

Treatment

All foreign bodies, once detected, should be immediately removed by suitably experienced staff in a properly equipped hospital. It is essential to have suitably designed forceps for grasping the foreign body so as to minimize mucosal damage. Occasionally a formal thoracic operation may be necessary.

Swallowed foreign bodies

The variety of swallowed foreign bodies is legion (Fig. 2). However, the majority are coins, fish bones, meat bones and lumps of meat. Children frequently swallow a handful of coins at a time. In adults, ingestion of foreign bodies is more likely if the patient uses dentures. These prevent adequate chewing and with a full upper plate there is some sensory deprivation.

Sites of impaction

Fish bones tend to lodge in the oropharynx (posterior tongue, vallecula and tonsil). Most other foreign bodies will tend to impact at sites of narrowing of the pharyngo-oesophagus (Fig. 3). These are piriform fossa and postcricoid region, particularly at the level of the cricopharyngeus muscle. The aorta and left main bronchus constrict the mid-oesophagus and there is a relatively reduced diameter at the gastro-oesophageal junction.

Clinical features

Most patients give a reliable history of foreign body ingestion. If lodged in the mouth or pharynx, localization is possible with the patient frequently pointing to the side affected. Symptoms are felt in the midline if the object has

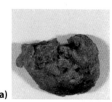

(a)

(b)

(c)

Fig. 2 (left)
A selection of swallowed foreign bodies. (a) A large piece of meat that was impacted at the gastro-oesophageal junction. **(b)** A lamb bone removed from the hypopharynx. **(c)** A piece of chicken bone removed from the postcricoid region. The two crowns were dislodged by the rigid oesophagoscope.

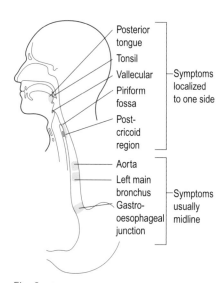

Fig. 3 **Sites of impaction of swallowed foreign bodies.**

passed beyond the postcricoid region. An impacted foreign body in the pharyngo-oesophagus will produce dramatic acute dysphagia, with difficulty in swallowing even saliva. Other symptoms such as otalgia, neck tenderness and fever are serious features and may indicate a rupture of the oesophagus. The presence of neck emphysema is indicative of a rupture of the pharyngo-oesophagus.

Visualization of foreign bodies

Most foreign bodies in the mouth and pharynx can be identified with the use of a head mirror and routine instruments, e.g. tongue depressors and laryngeal mirrors. The specific sites outlined in Figure 3 should be inspected. Fish bones frequently lodge in the tonsil and only a tiny length may project above the surface lining.

An oesophageal foreign body will be out of sight to routine examination, but commonly is associated with pooling of saliva in the piriform fossae. X-rays may be unhelpful because only radio-opaque objects will be visualized (Fig. 4), but soft tissue changes can be indicative.

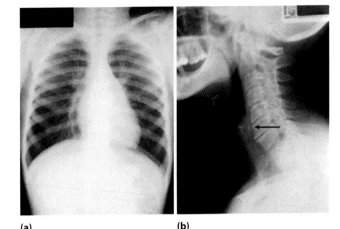

(a) **(b)**

Fig. 4 **Radio-opaque bodies that have been swallowed. (a)** A coin located in the lower oesophagus. **(b)** A lamb bone in the hypopharynx.

Treatment

Generally, a foreign body visualized on routine examination can be removed with angled forceps. This is especially true of fish bones lodged in the tonsil or vallecula. It is kinder to apply topical anaesthesia prior to removal. All sharp foreign bodies should be extracted at the earliest opportunity due to the risk of perforation. In patients with persistent symptoms, despite normal examination and radiology, it is necessary to exclude a foreign body, so pharyngo-oesophagoscopy should be performed.

A food bolus impacted in the oesophagus may be left for 6–12 hours and sedatives can be administered to the patient to encourage the bolus to pass on. If bone or other solid objects are involved, they should be removed at the earliest opportunity as there is an increased risk of perforation.

In adults with pharyngo-oesophageal foreign bodies it is important to exclude underlying pathology (Fig. 5). This is particularly so in the lower oesophagus and in the region of the gastro-oesophageal junction.

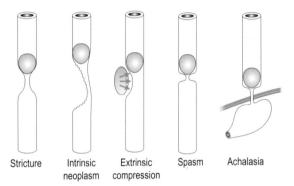

Stricture   Intrinsic   Extrinsic   Spasm   Achalasia
             neoplasm   compression

Fig. 5 **The potential underlying causes of impaction of a swallowed foreign body in adults.**

Management after pharyngo-oesophagoscopy

It is vital to ensure that a proper regimen of patient care is given after a pharyngo-oesophagoscopy, whether a foreign body was found and removed or not.

Oesophageal rupture

In all pharyngo-oesophageal endoscopies there is a risk of perforating the lumen. The cardinal features of an oesophageal rupture are shown in Table 1, and are due to food, bacteria and digestive juices contaminating the periluminal areas. The precise combination of clinical features is dependent on whether the perforation is in the cervical or thoracic oesophagus. Cardiorespiratory features predominate in the latter site.

Treatment of oesophageal rupture

Oesophageal rupture, either spontaneous or after endoscopy, requires urgent attention to avoid the 50% mortality associated with a treatment delay of 24 hours. The patient is kept nil by mouth. An intravenous line should be inserted to provide a measure of central venous pressure and parenteral feeding. Broad-spectrum antibiotics are required intravenously. A contrast swallow may allow visualization of the site of a leak.

Surgical intervention will be required in a deteriorating situation or for surgical drainage of abscesses.

Table 1 **Symptoms and signs of oesophageal perforation**
Pain in neck, chest and back
Pyrexia
Tachycardia and dyspnoea
Surgical emphysema: clinical and radiological

Foreign bodies

- Inhaled foreign bodies lodged in the larynx may be immediately fatal.
- Cough and wheezing developing in a previously well child should alert the clinician to the presence of an inhaled foreign body.
- A time lapse of days to months may occur between inhalation of foreign bodies and clinical symptoms: dependent on the nature of the object, i.e. vegetable or non-vegetable.
- Swallowed foreign bodies located in the mouth and pharynx generally produce ipsilateral symptoms.
- Oesophageal foreign bodies are usually localized in the midline.
- A good headlight, simple instruments and angled forceps will enable most foreign bodies in the mouth and pharynx to be removed.
- Solid impacted oesophageal foreign bodies may pass spontaneously.
- Exclude underlying pathology in foreign bodies impacted in the oesophagus.
- Educate all medical and nursing staff in the features of a pharyngo-oesophageal perforation after endoscopic examination.

ENT aspects of HIV infection

The human immunodeficiency viruses (HIV) are a group of retroviruses which are characterized by their ability to impair immunological defences against infection and neoplasia. Manifestations of HIV infection in the ear, nose and throat are very common, occurring in about 40% of HIV patients. Infection with HIV may lead to the condition known as AIDS (acquired immune deficiency syndrome).

Incidence and aetiology

Although HIV is primarily a disease affecting homosexuals, it is also known to occur in heterosexuals, bisexuals and those receiving infected blood products, e.g. haemophiliacs and i.v. drug users. The virus is transmitted via a breech in the lining epithelium. Transfer can be through blood, semen or maternal milk in the suckling. The symptoms and signs are related to the effect of HIV on the cellular immune system. In particular, the virus primarily affects T lymphocytes, thus reducing cell-mediated immunity.

Clinical features

Persistent generalized lymphadenopathy (PGL)

PGL is an early feature of HIV infection. It presents as persistent, firm, non-tender lymph glands in several sites, often accompanied by fever, night sweats, weight loss, fatigue and diarrhoea. The cervical glands are frequently involved. PGL is diagnosed if at least two sites, other than the inguinal region, have glands of 1 cm or greater in diameter present for at least 3 months, and in the absence of a specific factor (e.g. acute viral illness or immunization) that could cause lymphadenopathy. The patient is frequently asymptomatic.

AIDS-related complex (ARC)

ARC is a later stage in the disease progression. It is a group of symptoms and signs in the absence of other opportunistic infection and neoplasia (e.g. Kaposi's sarcoma). Symptoms include malaise, fevers and night sweats, weight loss and unexplained diarrhoea. Many of the clinical signs of ARC may present as ENT manifestations (Table 1).

Full-blown AIDS

Full blown AIDS is defined as opportunistic infections and tumours

Table 1 **Clinical signs of ARC**
Oral candidiasis (Fig. 1, p. 72)
Oral leukoplakia (hairy leukoplakia)
PGL
Seborrhoeic dermatitis (scalp and external ear canal)
Rhinosinusitis

indicative of cellular immune deficiency in previously normal individuals with no known cause for immune deficiency. The classic opportunistic infection is in the lungs and is caused by *Pneumocystis carinii* (Fig. 1). Candidal infection of the mouth and extending into the oesophagus is not infrequent, and results in severe dysphagia. Rhinosinusitis, causing postnasal discharge and sinofacial discomfort, is very common in AIDS. PGL affecting lymphoid tissue in the nasopharynx can cause blockage of the Eustachian tube and subsequent secretory otitis media. Intraoral ulceration in AIDS may be due to herpes virus infection. It is similar in appearance to the usual benign variety, but does not resolve spontaneously. Of the neoplasias, the most common is Kaposi's sarcoma. These appear as small, bluish, painless skin lesions and the head, neck and oral cavity may be involved (Figs 2&3). Other tumours include non-Hodgkin's lymphoma (B-cell type) and squamous cell carcinoma. Parotid enlargement can be an early presenting sign of HIV disease.

Management

Treatment is mainly symptomatic in ARC and directed toward the secondary manifestations of AIDS. Opportunistic infections require antibiotics, e.g. antifungal agents for mucosal candidiasis. Long-term prophylaxis is required to prevent relapse. Rhinosinusitis may require drainage of the sinus, and secretory otitis media the insertion of a ventilating tube. Herpetic oral ulceration is controlled with aciclovir treatment.

Kaposi's sarcoma, if on the skin surface, may need no treatment. Intraoral lesions can be excised or treated with radiotherapy. B-cell lymphomas require conventional chemotherapeutic regimens.

Specific therapy to treat the underlying defect of the cellular immune system is not available. Antiretroviral triple therapy is usually commenced when there is a low CD4 lymphocyte count, high viral load or

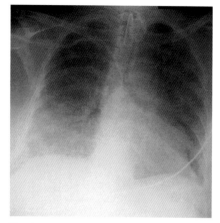

Fig. 1　*Pneumocystic carinii* **lung infection.**

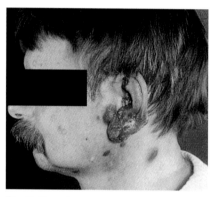

Fig. 2　**Kaposi's sarcoma affecting the skin of the head and neck.**

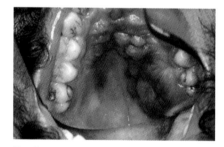

Fig. 3　**Kaposi's sarcoma presenting in the oral cavity.**

AIDS presentation. As a result of this therapy, patients live longer with HIV infection and have a higher quality of life during the course of the disease.

ENT aspects of HIV infection

- AIDS is caused by HIV and affects the cellular immune system.
- The cervical glands may be involved in primary HIV infection.
- Rhinosinusitis is the commonest ENT manifestation.
- Extranodal lymphomas and squamous carcinoma may develop in the oral cavity or oropharynx

Head and Neck Neoplasia

Basic concepts

Head and neck tumours include a wide spectrum of pathologies with different patterns of behaviour. The complex anatomy of this region makes their management difficult as therapy may result in disruption of speech, swallowing and cosmesis. Patients with head and neck cancer need to be treated in specialist (tertiary) cancer centres by specialist multidisciplinary teams (MDT).

Squamous cell carcinoma of the upper aerodigestive tract accounts for over 90% of tumours in this region (Table 1).

Management of head and neck cancer is dependent on histological diagnosis, staging and grading of the tumour. The patient's wishes are equally important factors in determining therapy. Some patients may not be fit for aggressive curative treatment and others may refuse treatment. The head and neck oncologist uses surgery, radiotherapy and chemotherapy as treatment modalities. In general, early cancers are treated with single modality therapy and advanced cancers require combined modality. A treatment algorithm for head and neck cancer is shown in Figure 1.

Aetilogical factors

Cancer develops through a complex multifactorial process (Fig. 2). The majority of head and neck cancers result from exposure to carcinogens, mainly via tobacco. Chewing tobacco is also carcinogenic and associated with mouth cancer. Alcohol appears to act synergistically with smoking. Betel nut, which is widely chewed in the Indian subcontinent, is a strong carcinogen for mouth cancer, hence the very high incidence of oral cancer in this region. Exposure to ionizing radiation is implicated in thyroid cancer and sarcomas. Oncogenic viruses such as human papilloma virus (HPV) are known to induce tumours in squamous epithelium. Epstein–Barr

virus (EBV) is associated with nasopharyngeal cancer and Burkitt's lymphoma. Heavy metals, such as nickel or chromium, and hardwood dust exposure are important occupational carcinogens. Severe chronic dental caries is thought to predispose to mouth cancer.

Genetic factors also predispose to cancer. Multiple endocrine neoplasia (MEN) is an inherited condition associated with medullary thyroid cancer (MTC) and caused by a specific gene mutation.

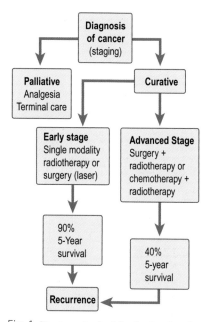

Fig. 1 **Treatment principles for head and neck cancer.**

Premalignant conditions in head and neck cancer

Head and neck cancer may develop de novo but in a significant proportion of cases premalignant conditions exist long before the tumour develops. These lesions arise due to chronic exposure to carcinogens. Dysplasia is the pathological term to describe changes in the cell structure and epithelium architecture which predispose to cancer. Dysplasia ranges from mild, moderate, severe to carcinoma-in-situ. The management of dysplastic lesions depends upon their size, severity and location. Lifestyle changes are very important: if exposure to the carcinogen is removed, the dysplastic lesion may resolve. Surgery is used to remove localized premalignant lesions. Radiotherapy is useful in diffuse dysplasia. Retinoids have been used also in oral dysplasia. New diagnostic screening mouthwashes are also available to detect premalignant lesions.

Clinical manifestations of premalignant conditions are leukoplakia (white patch) or erythroplasia (red patch) which may affect the mucosa (Figs 3 & 4). These often present as superficial lesions and should be biopsied to determine grade of dysplasia.

Lichen planus
Erosive lichen planus of the oral cavity (Fig. 5) may progress to cancer. The common form of lichen planus, which is benign, is located in a symmetrical

Table 1 **Head and neck cancer subtypes**
Squamous cell carcinoma
Lymphoma (Hodgkin's & non-Hodgkin's)
Adenocarcinoma
Adenoid cystic carcinoma
Thyroid carcinoma (follicular, papillary, medullary, anaplastic)
Sarcomas

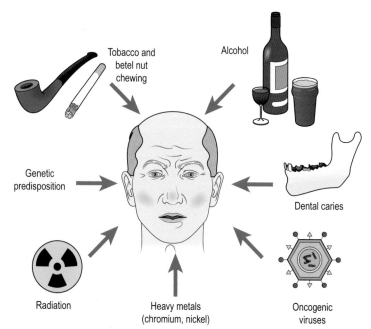

Fig. 2 **Aetiological factors in the development of head and neck neoplasia.**

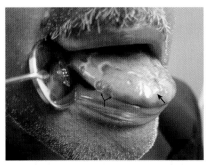

Fig. 3 **Leukoplakia (↖) and erythroplasia (Ⲩ) of the oral tongue.** Note the staining from betel nut chewing on the contralateral side of the tongue.

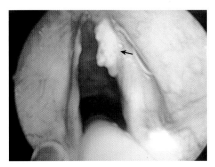

Fig. 4 **Leukoplakia of the larynx in a heavy smoker.** The right vocal cord is affected by dysplastic epithelium (↑).

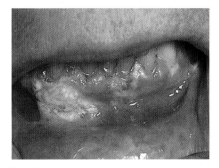

Fig. 5 **Erosive lichen planus.**

distribution on the buccal mucosa and tongue. The erosive variety appears in the floor of the mouth. Biopsy is mandatory to identify the type of lichen planus and to distinguish it from leucoplakia.

Principles of treatment

The treatment options in head and neck neoplasia include:

■ radiotherapy ± chemotherapy
■ surgical excision
■ terminal care (p. 116).

The preferred modalities, either singularly or in combination, can only be determined by patient assessment, histological information and the extent of the local and regional disease. The majority of head and neck malignancies require primary radiotherapy followed by salvage surgery for recurrent and residual disease (RRD). In advanced disease, treatment will be palliation.

Radiotherapy

Ionizing radiation destroys cancer cells by preventing their division. Irradiation sources include X-rays, gamma and beta rays. More recently, fast neutrons have been employed, but with disappointing results. Since all tissue will absorb radiation, it is important to minimize unacceptable damage. This is achieved by accurate localization and by fractionating the radiation dosage.

Unfortunately, two structures, the lens of the eye and the spinal cord, are highly sensitive to irradiation. Exposure of these two organs is avoided by accurate planning of the radiotherapy fields (based on clinical examination and CT/MRI imaging). A specific mask is constructed to keep the head and neck steady during therapy.

The majority of patients will develop radiation reactions in normal tissue. The skin will invariably show some evidence of treatment (Fig. 6). Mucous membrane reactions tend to occur very early, with erythema and ulceration and may be so severe that nasogastric feeding is required. Fungal infections, particularly by *Candida*, often compound the mucositis and are not uncommon in the debilitated patient. Prophylactic care with antifungals and anti-inflammatory rinses may be required.

Chemotherapy

Chemotherapy is rarely used as the sole modality of treatment. It has traditionally been reserved for patients presenting with advanced disease or in recurrent or residual disease after radiotherapy and surgery. Trials are ongoing to document if chemotherapy employed in synchrony with radiation confers any increase in survival over radiotherapy alone.

The major side effect of chemotherapeutic agents is their depressive action on haemopoiesis.

This toxicity is increased in the presence of abnormal liver and renal function.

Surgery

Surgical excision will result in some degree of cosmetic and functional deficit. The deficit is related to the extent of ablation and the availability of reconstructive manoeuvres. Resection should be with a 2 cm margin of clearance from the tumour edge. Reconstructive options include local and regional pedicled flaps and microvascular free grafts.

Terminal care

Some patients have no prospect of cure due to advanced disease or residual or recurrent disease. The dying phase is usually protracted. In order to be able to deal with such situations in a humane manner, the concept of terminal care has evolved. This provides the physical and psychological support for patients in the terminal stage of their life (see p. 116).

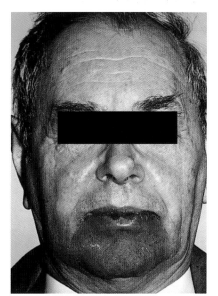

Fig. 6 **Radiotherapy skin reaction.** The mucous membrane of the lip is severely ulcerated.

Basic concepts

■ Head and neck malignancy uncommonly produces distant metastases.
■ Tobacco and alcohol are the major aetiological factors in development of head and neck malignancy.
■ Any neck mass should only the biopsied after a full examination of the upper air and food passages has been performed to exclude a primary neoplastic process.
■ The use of radiotherapy is limited by sensitivity of surrounding normal tissues, particularly damage to the lens of the eye and spinal cord.
■ Severe radiation reactions may necessitate a temporary halt to the course of radiotherapy.
■ Chemotherapeutic agents appear to enhance the effect of radiotherapy, but their present role is not yet fully evaluated.

Neck lumps — Introduction

Many neck swellings may be diagnosed after a comprehensive history and a thorough clinical examination of the head and neck. Further evaluation with imaging, endoscopy and biopsy will be required in some instances. It is inappropriate to resort to biopsy until a full evaluation of potential local and distant diagnoses has been undertaken. An incorrect biopsy technique of a neck lump may compromise the prognosis of a patient with metastatic neck disease.

It is useful to consider separately the diagnosis of neck lumps in children and adults. The '80:20 rule' applies to malignant and benign causes of neck masses (Fig. 1). In the adult it must be remembered that metastatic neck disease may occur from structures below the clavicle (Table 1).

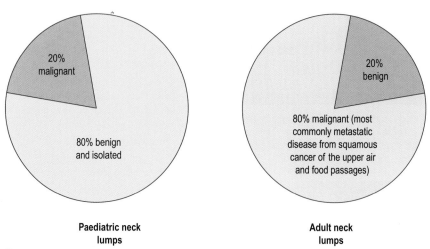

Fig. 1 **The '80:20' rule applied to neck lumps.**

Table 1 **Intraclavicular sites of malignancy that may cause neck lumps by metastatic spread**	
Lung	Kidney
Breast	Prostate
Stomach	Uterus
Pancreas	

Clinical history and examination

In addition to a routine history, specific questions must be posed. The '20:40 rule' is useful in considering the diagnostic possibilities of a neck lump (Table 2).

The presence of pain is a helpful clue to diagnosis. Inflamed tissue, e.g. the lymph nodes, will be tender. Salivary gland calculi may present with recurrent pain and swelling, especially during eating. Congenital lesions such as branchial and thyroglossal cysts may present as painful neck lumps. It is important to establish whether the lump is increasing, decreasing or static in size. The level of tobacco and alcohol intake should be determined.

The primary head and neck sites of malignancy may give rise to very specific symptoms including:

- dysphagia (pharyngo-oesophagus)
- dysphonia (larynx and hypopharynx).

Earache may be referred from neoplastic lesions in the upper food passages (Fig. 4, p. 13). Referred otalgia is a poor prognostic sign in head and neck neoplasia.

Table 2 **The '20:40 rule' applied to neck lumps**	
Age (years)	Possible causes of neck lump
Less than 20	Inflammatory neck nodes (e.g. due to tonsilllitis)
	Congenital lesions (e.g. thyroglossal cysts, brachial cyst, midline dermoid, cystic hygroma)
	Lymphoma
20–40	Salivary gland pathology (calculus, infection, tumour)
	Thyroid pathology (tumour, thyroiditis, goitre, lymphoma)
	Chronic infection (tuberculosis, HIV)
Greater than 40	Primary or secondary malignant disease

In the presence of a neck lump, any weight loss is significant and implies the presence of malignant disease. If associated with dysphagia, the site is usually in the upper digestive tract, but particularly of the pharyngo-oesophageal region.

Certain systemic symptoms may also give clues to the aetiology of a neck lump. Malaise is a feature of lymphoma and tuberculosis. Nocturnal fevers and pruritus are also common in lymphoma.

It is important to perform a thorough examination of the head and neck, especially the upper aerodigestive tract, as well as looking for other lumps, e.g. in the liver, spleen or axillae. The scalp should be carefully examined, as a primary malignancy in this site is commonly overlooked as a cause of metastatic neck disease. The precise features of the lump should be noted and, if laterally sited, its position in the triangles of the neck accurately described (Fig. 2). This approach is useful as an aid to remembering structures located in the triangles which may give

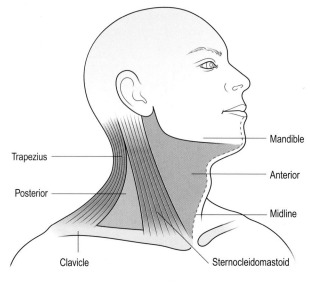

Fig. 2 **The triangle of the neck.** The sternocleidomastoid divides the neck into two triangles, the boundaries of which are shown. The anterior triangle contains lymph nodes, submandibular gland, tail of the parotid and the carotid bifurcation. The posterior triangle contains lymph nodes and the spinal accessory nerve.

rise to pathology. A mass in the midline is most frequently of thyroid origin. Nasopharyngeal carcinoma may present as unilateral or bilateral metastatic nodes in the posterior triangle of the neck. An isolated mass in the supraclavicular region is likely to be metastatic disease from sites below the clavicle (Table 1).

Multiple neck lumps are most likely to be lymph nodes. There are over 100 lymph nodes on each side of the neck, although they tend to be confined to relatively discrete areas rather than evenly distributed (Fig. 3).

Palpation of a neck lump may reveal the presence of pulsation, e.g. carotid body tumours. It is important to determine that this pulsation is not transmitted from arteries in the neck. A pulsatile neck lump should be auscultated to detect the presence of a bruit.

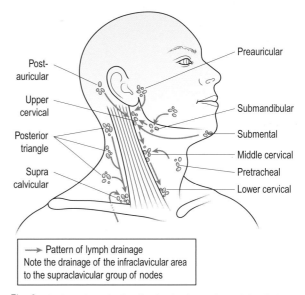

Fig. 3 **The lymph node distribution in the neck, and the drainage pattern.**

Investigations
At a minimum the special investigations should incorporate:

- a full blood count
- sedimentation rate
- chest X-ray (Fig. 4).

Biopsy of a neck lump
The diagnosis of a neck lump may be dependent on biopsy. This should only be undertaken after extensive investigations to exclude pathology in potential primary head and neck sites. This would generally include a fine needle aspiration of the mass for cytological assessment. Examination under general anaesthesia of the upper aerodigestive tract may be required. If both aspiration cytology and a full examination under anaesthesia are negative, an open excisional biopsy should be performed, with a view to proceeding to neck dissection.

With this systematic approach, many neoplasms can be diagnosed without recourse to open biopsy, avoiding the danger of implanting in the neck skin.

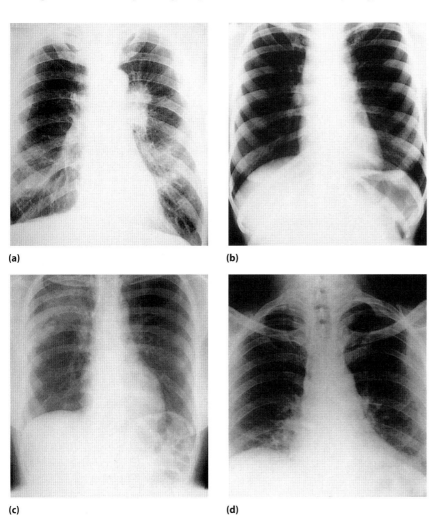

(a)

(b)

(c)

(d)

Fig. 4 **The value of a plain chest X-ray in the investigation of neck lumps. (a)** A carcinoma of the lung (left hilum) may give rise to metastatic neck disease. **(b)** Lymphoma in the neck is frequently associated with disease in the chest (widened mediastinum). **(c)** Pulmonary (right apex) and cervical tuberculosis is now rare. **(d)** A cervical rib (right) may be mistaken for a pathological neck lump.

Neck lumps – introduction

- Never biopsy a neck lump without a prior thorough ENT examination of the upper air and food passages.
- Remember the 80:20 percentage and the 20:40 age rules in the diagnosis of neck lumps.
- Do not forget infraclavicular sites for metastatic neck lumps, particularly adenocarcinoma.
- Palpate the salivary and thyroid glands and listen for any overlying vascular bruits.
- Multiple neck lumps are almost certainly lymph nodes.
- Fine needle aspiration cytology may assist in diagnosis.
- Avoid incisional biopsy of a neck lump; if malignant disease is present there is a risk of implantation.
- It is normal in children to have easily palpable lymph nodes in the neck.
- Do not overlook HIV infection as a cause of lymphadenopathy.

Neck lumps — Paediatric conditions

In the paediatric age group (<20 years of age), the majority of neck lumps encountered are benign. They are commonly located anterior to the sternomastoid muscle in the anterior triangle of the neck. An isolated neck lump located in the posterior triangle has a high likelihood of being malignant. The '80:20 rule' is useful in assessing the diagnostic possibilities (Fig. 1, p. 90).

For diagnostic and descriptive purposes, neck lumps can be described by their position: midline or lateral.

Midline neck lumps

Thyroglossal cyst
The commonest midline mass (Fig. 1) in children is a congenital cyst of the thyroglossal duct. Embryologically, the cyst can arise at any site along the route of the thyroglossal duct, extending from the tongue (foramen caecum) to the thyroid gland.

The thyroglossal cyst is most commonly located below the hyoid bone, and moves both on swallowing and tongue protrusion (Figs. 1 & 2). Most cysts are asymptomatic, apart from the presence of a lump, but infection will be associated with pain and swelling. Treatment is by excision, which should include the central portion of the body of the hyoid bone to prevent recurrences. A wedge of tongue muscle is resected with the thyroglossal duct behind the hyoid.

Dermoid cyst
Dermoid cysts usually present as submental swellings in the midline. They are dermal remnants occurring along the lines of fusion in the embryo. These cysts are lined by epidermis and may contain hair, teeth and squamous debris. They tend not to move on swallowing or tongue protrusion. Dermoid cysts should be excised.

Miscellaneous lumps
Other midline lumps are rare in children. Chondromas of the cartilaginous structures of the larynx are hard to palpation, and move on swallowing. Treatment is by excision. Occasionally a pyramidal lobe of the thyroid may present as a midline lump. An ultrasound and isotope scan will reveal the underlying cause. Lymph nodes located in the midline of the neck may enlarge secondary to infection or neoplasia.

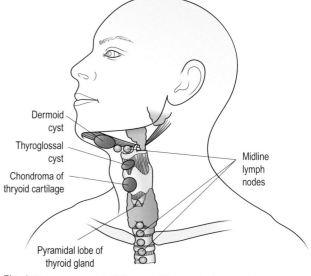

Fig. 1 **Some causes of midline neck lumps in the paediatric age group.**

Labels: Dermoid cyst; Thyroglossal cyst; Chondroma of thyroid cartilage; Pyramidal lobe of thyroid gland; Midline lymph nodes

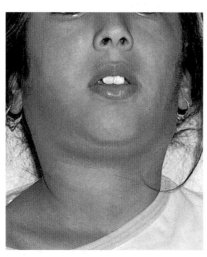

Fig. 2 **A thyroglossal cyst.**

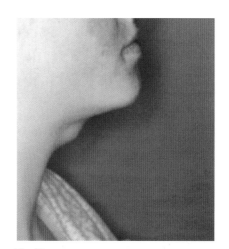

Fig. 3 **Bilateral parotid enlargement due to mumps.**

Lateral neck lumps (Table 1)

Inflammatory conditions
Enlarged infected lymph glands of the neck are the commonest cause of lateral neck lumps in children. An infective aetiology is accompanied at some stage by tender enlargement. Multiple palpable, non-tender nodes are a normal feature in many children.

The primary areas for infection in the head and neck should be carefully inspected and include the skin and scalp in addition to the oral cavity, oropharynx and nasopharynx. The commonest infections are of the upper respiratory tract, tonsils and teeth. Resolution of infective lymph nodes is rapid as the primary infection settles. Persistent lymphadenopathy should be re-evaluated.

Mumps
Enlargement of the parotid glands, due to the mumps virus, is extremely common. It is usually a bilateral disease, but unilateral cases can occur (Fig. 3). The child has constitutional symptoms of malaise and pyrexia. Rare cases may be complicated by orchitis and encephalitis. Treatment is symptomatic.

Tuberculosis
Tuberculosis of the cervical lymph nodes is uncommon. Tuberculous nodes are multiple and coalesce, and

Table 1 **Causes of lateral neck lumps in children**	
Infective	Cervical lymphadenitis
	Mumps
	Tuberculosis
Congenital	Branchial cysts
	Chemodectoma
	Cystic hygroma
	Haemangioma
Neoplastic	
Primary	Lymphoma
	Neuroblastoma
	Parotid malignancy
	Rhabdomyosarcomas
Secondary	Metastases — nasopharyngeal

may form a discharging sinus (Fig. 4). Most cases have associated pulmonary tuberculosis. Node biopsy is sometimes required for histological confirmation of diagnosis. Treatment is by combination chemotherapy.

Congenital conditions
Most solitary lateral neck masses in the paediatric age group are congenital in origin.

Branchial arch cysts
Branchial arch anomalies giving rise to branchial cysts are uncommon. First branchial arch cysts are rare and located anterior to the tragus. True branchial cysts are more frequently encountered and invariably located in the anterior triangle just in front of the sternomastoid (Fig. 5). The aetiology is believed to be cystic degeneration in a lymph node. Most of these cysts are lined by lymphoid tissue so that pain and swelling may be experienced with upper respiratory infections. Where a second arch fistula is present a tract may extend to the pharynx, and this must be excised together with the cyst.

Cystic hygromas
Cystic hygromas are anomalies of the lymph channels and present as lateral neck swellings. They are soft and irregular, and usually present at birth (Fig. 6). Typically, the hygroma enlarges during crying and the Valsalva manoeuvre. They transilluminate brilliantly. Most cystic hygromas have to be removed due to continued enlargement, particularly as they may encroach onto the major airways. Excision is difficult, as this benign lesion encompasses structures such as the carotid arteries and facial nerve.

Chemodectomas and haemangiomas
Chemodectomas (glomus tumours) are extremely rare benign tumours

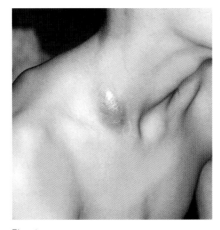
Fig. 4 **Tuberculous neck nodes about to discharge through the skin.**

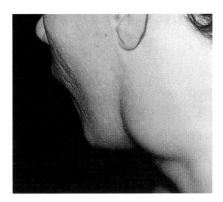
Fig. 5 **A lateral neck swelling due to a branchial cyst.**

arising from the carotid bulb in the region of the carotid bifurcations. They are pulsatile, and a bruit is audible with a stethoscope. Palpation reveals movement in the lateral but not vertical plane. Magnetic resonance imaging confirms the diagnosis. Surgical treatment will be required in the young age group. In the elderly they may be left untreated as the tumour is extremely slow growing and the risk of metastases is very small.

Haemangiomas are seen in the neonatal period. They are extremely rare and many regress as the child matures. Treatment is required only if the lesion is enlarging and the patient is symptomatic.

Neoplasia
Neoplasia is usually due to primary cancer in the neck, but secondary metastatic disease, particularly from the nasopharynx, can present as an isolated neck lump.

Lymphoma of the Hodgkin's variety is common. It may present as a unilateral isolated lump in the neck (Fig. 7). After histological confirmation, a full evaluation will be required to stage the disease. Treatment is usually

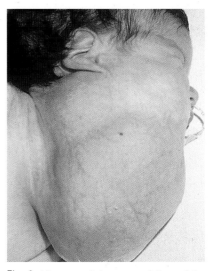
Fig. 6 **A large cystic hygroma of the neck in a neonate.**

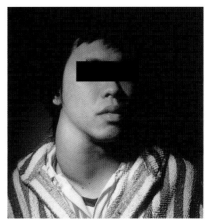
Fig. 7 **Swelling of the right neck due to lymphoma.**

radiotherapy in localized disease and chemotherapy with drug combinations in systemic lymphoma.

Rarer primary neoplasia include malignant parotid disease, rhabomyosarcomas and neuroblastomas.

Neck lumps – paediatric conditions

- 80% of neck lumps in children are benign and are located in the anterior triangle of the neck.

- 20% of neck lumps in children are malignant and are usually located in the posterior triangle of the neck.

- The commonest midline lump in children is the thyroglossal cyst. It moves on swallowing and with tongue protrusion.

- The commonest cause of multiple lateral neck lumps in children is cervical lymphadenopathy secondary to infection.

- The commonest isolated lateral neck lump in children is the branchial cyst.

Neck lumps — Adult conditions

The majority of adult neck lumps are malignant in origin, with metastatic squamous cell carcinoma from the upper aerodigestive tract being the commonest cause. Benign masses constitute 20% of the total.

Midline neck lumps

Thyroid masses

The thyroid gland is a hormonal gland lying in the midline of the neck at the level of the thyroid cartilage. It consists of a left and right lobe joined by an isthmus. Thyroid masses are common and a systematic approach to managing them should be adopted.

It is important to determine whether there is a goitre (diffuse bilateral thyroid enlargement) or a nodular (single) mass within the thyroid (Figs 1 & 2). Symptoms and signs of hyper-(overactive) and hypo-(underactive) thyroid disease should be sought (Table 1). Clinical examination should determine the size and nature of the thyroid mass. Thyroid enlargement may result in compression of either the trachea, causing stridor, or oesophagus,

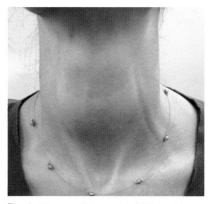

Fig. 1 **Woman with a goitre (diffuse thyroid enlargement).**

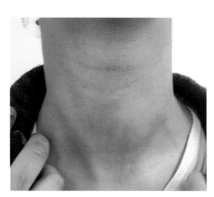

Fig. 2 **Woman with single left thyroid nodule.**

causing dysphagia. Common disorders to affect the thyroid gland include thyroiditis, multinodular goitre, follicular adenoma, thyroid carcinoma and lymphoma.

Investigations

Blood tests should determine thyroid status; a TSH test is the first-line investigation. Autoimmune thyroid antibodies should be measured along with thyroglobulin. Fine needle aspiration cytology (FNAC) should be undertaken to determine the cellular nature of any thyroid nodule. Ultrasound scanning is the first imaging of choice; it will determine whether the thyroid swelling is cystic or solid and will demonstrate whether multiple nodules are present. Ultrasound and FNAC can be combined to increase diagnostic yield. CT scanning is only indicated when tracheal compression or retrosternal extension is suspected (Fig. 3).

Management

Abnormal thyroid status must be controlled and this may involve drug treatment. Nodular thyroid swellings are usually managed by thyroid lobectomy. Goitres may need total thyroidectomy if they cause compressive symptoms.

Table 1 **Symptoms and signs of thyroid disease**		
Disease	**Symptoms**	**Signs**
Hyperthyroidism	Palpitations	Tachycardia (AF)
	Weight loss	Exophthalmos
	Agitation	Tremor
	Sweating	
Hypothyroidism	Tiredness	Bradycardia
	Weight gain	Loss of eyebrow
	Poor concentration	hair

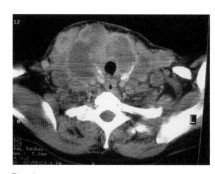

Fig. 3 **CT scan of neck with large goitre compressing the trachea.**

Thyroid cancer

Thyroid cancer is rare and accounts for only 1–2% of cancers in the UK. The majority present as solitary nodules in the thyroid gland, but only 10% of solitary nodules will turn out to be cancerous.

The common thyroid cancers are papillary, follicular, medullary and anaplastic. Management involves FNAC to diagnose the lesion, imaging and staging. Treatment comprises surgery (a total thyroidectomy) followed by radioiodine ablation. In general a 90% survival at 10 years can be expected with differentiated thyroid cancer.

Miscellaneous midline lumps

Thyroglossal cysts, midline dermoids and a prominent pyramidal lobe of the thyroid may all be causes of midline neck lumps in adults. These have been discussed elsewhere (p. 92).

Lateral neck lumps

Neoplasia

Any neck lump appearing for the first time in an adult over 40 years of age should be treated as metastatic cancer until proven otherwise (Table 2). Secondary neck disease from malignancy in the upper aerodigestive tract is very common. The patient frequently gives a long history of alcohol and tobacco abuse. The possibility of a supraclavicular neck mass being metastatic disease from sites below the clavicle should not be overlooked (Table 1, p. 90).

Unilateral painless parotid masses are likely to be neoplastic, the commonest lesion being the benign pleomorphic adenoma. Malignant parotid tumours may cause pain and facial weakness due to involvement of the facial nerve (p. 113). Hodgkin's and non-Hodgkin's lymphoma may initially present as an isolated lateral neck lump. However, disease progression leads to multiple matted neck lumps.

Certain tumours of neural crest origin may present as lateral neck lumps in the adult. These include carotid body tumours, glomus vagale and neurofibromas of the vagus nerve. Multiple neurofibromata (café au lait skin pigmentation and cutaneous and neural tumours) may be associated with von Recklinghausen's disease.

Table 2 Causes of a lateral neck lump in adults

Type	Condition
Neoplasia	Primary cancer
	Lymphoma
	Neurogenic (schwannoma, chemodectoma)
	Metastatic cancer
	Lymph node metastasis from head and neck sites
Infection	Glandular fever
	HIV
	Tuberculosis
	Parotitis (mumps)
Autoimmune	Sjögren's syndrome
Miscellaneous	Sarcoidosis
	Branchial cyst
Normal variants	Transverse process of 2nd cervical vertebra (C2)
	Enlongated styloid process
	Normal or cervical rib
	Tortuous, atherosclerotic carotid artery

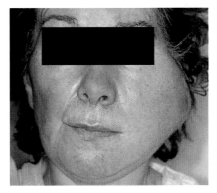
Fig. 4 **A unilateral parotid swelling caused by a bacterial parotitis.**

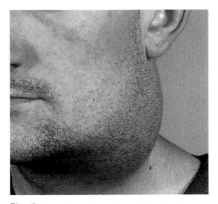
Fig. 5 **An external neck swelling due to infection in the parapharyngeal space.**

Inflammatory conditions
Glandular fever is a common infection in young adults and invariably presents as a sore throat, similar to an acute streptococcal tonsillitis, with bilateral tender enlargement of cervical nodes. Severe cases may also have hepatosplenomegaly and haematological abnormalities. The diagnosis is confirmed by the presence of atypical monocytes in the peripheral blood and a positive serological test to Epstein–Barr virus antibodies (Paul–Bunnell or Monospot tests).

Acute parotitis, either bacterial or viral, may cause neck swelling (Fig. 4). The diagnosis is usually straightforward – provided the full anatomical extent of the parotid is appreciated, including the deep lobe which may enlarge into the oropharynx. An infection of the parapharyngeal space of the neck, usually from dental or oropharyngeal infections, may produce a significant neck swelling in association with a mass in the throat (Fig. 5).

Tuberculosis in the cervical nodes is uncommon in Europe but very frequent in the developing countries. If not associated with pulmonary tuberculosis, an excisional biopsy may be required to confirm the diagnosis.

Sjögren's syndrome
Sjögren's syndrome is a triad of xerostomia (dry mouth); keratoconjunctivitis sicca (dry eye) and a systemic autoimmune disease, e.g. rheumatoid arthritis or scleroderma. Parotid enlargement, usually bilateral, is due to lymphocytic infiltration, and the gland shows a reduction in saliva formation. The lacrimal glands are similarly involved, which results in reduced or absent tear formation. Autoantibodies are present in the peripheral blood. A buccal labial biopsy with histological grading is the diagnostic investigation.

Treatment is symptomatic, with the provision of artificial tears and saliva. However, these patients require long-term follow-up, as a small percentage will develop lymphoma in the parotid gland.

Miscellaneous lateral lumps
Sarcoidosis
Sarcoidosis in the neck rarely occurs without mediastinal disease. If hilar involvement is absent, diagnosis is made by biopsy of the neck lump which reveals the typical non-caseating granulomas. The finding of raised serum angiotensin-converting enzyme levels is diagnostic.

HIV infection
The primary infection with the human immunodeficiency virus (HIV) may produce prodromal symptoms similar to glandular fever (p. 86). Persistent lymphadenopathy syndrome (PLS) is seen in the chronic stage of infection with HIV, with lymph nodes in the neck being commonly enlarged.

Normal variants
Certain normal bony and cartilaginous structures in the neck may be palpable in some patients and mistaken for lumps (Fig. 6). The lateral process of the axis (C2) Is frequently palpable and tender if slight pressure is applied. These features may only be demonstrated on one side of the neck. The styloid process may be elongated and ossified, and therefore palpable as it runs just anterior from the mastoid to the mandible. Normal ribs and, occasionally, an asymptomatic cervical rib may be palpated deep in the supraclavicular fossa. A tortuous atherosclerotic carotid artery in a thin elderly person may be mistaken for a neck mass. It may not be pulsatile, but a bruit is usually audible on auscultation.

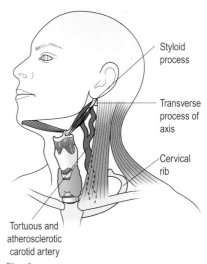
Fig. 6 **Normal variants that can mimic a lateral neck lump in adults.**

Neck lumps – adult conditions

- Thyroid lesions are the commonest cause of midline lumps in adults.
- The commonest lateral neck lump in adults is metastatic malignant disease, usually squamous cell carcinoma from a primary site in the head and neck.
- The symptoms and signs of acute infection with HIV mimic the clinical features of glandular fever.

Neck lumps — Management of malignant lumps

In some patients a neck mass may be a lymph node affected by infection, lymphoma or metastatic carcinoma, rather than the specific neck diseases discussed on previous pages.

The general management of such patients is outlined in Figure 1. A full ENT evaluation will include inspection, radiology and possible biopsy of primary sites in the head and neck. If the primary sites are clear, fine needle aspiration cytology (FNAC) may assist in the diagnosis. Otherwise, the mass must be biopsied by excision. Incisional biopsies carry the risk of producing implantation of malignant cells in skin with a poorer prognostic outlook.

The diagnosis of an inflammatory or lymphomatous process in a lymph node will allow appropriate therapy in the former, and staging and eventual treatment strategies in the latter. The general management of metastatic head and neck carcinoma is discussed below.

Metastatic cervical nodes

Metastatic cervical nodes are clinically assessed and then classified according to the UICC/AJC criteria (Table 1). Since the classification is clinically based, it is subject to observer variation. Additionally, it is not feasible to decide whether a palpable node does in fact contain metastatic cancer or is merely enlarged due to infection. The implication in the classification is that prognosis deteriorates from N1 through to N3 stages. More recently it appears that the level of metastatic disease in the neck is a better prognostic indicator than the mere presence of palpable nodes. Inferiorly placed neck disease has the worst prognosis, with supraclavicular node involvement having the least favourable 5-year survival.

The treatment of metastatic cervical nodes depends to a large degree on whether the primary disease in the head or neck, or in distant sites, has been uncovered. As a rule, surgery in the form of a radical neck dissection is advocated for metastatic neck disease (Fig. 2). This procedure attempts to remove all lymph node-bearing elements in the anterior and posterior triangle between the prevertebral fascia and platysma. Radiotherapy may be

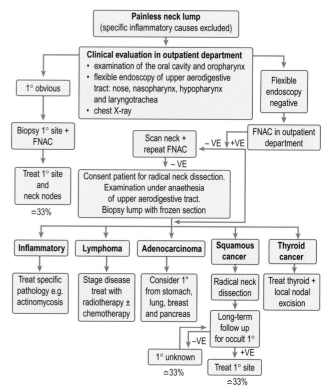

Fig. 1 **Management of an isolated neck lump.**

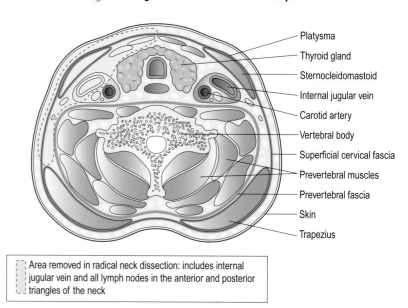

Area removed in radical neck dissection: includes internal jugular vein and all lymph nodes in the anterior and posterior triangles of the neck

Fig. 2 **Principles of the radical neck dissection for metastatic neck disease.**

employed in occult and small nodal metastases, and in palliation of fungating lesions.

N0: Clinically negative neck nodes

Impalpable lymph nodes involved in metastatic disease are called 'occult nodes'. There are certain sites in the head and neck, with a rich and frequently decussating lymphatic supply, in which metastatic nodal disease is highly probable (Table 2).

Although it would be logical therefore to consider performing an elective radical neck dissection in occult neck disease, such a policy shows little benefit. It appears that in selected

Table 1 **Classification of regional lymph nodes affected by metastatic carcinoma**	
Classification (UICC/AJC)	Clinical assessment
N0	No regional nodes palpable
N1	Mobile ipsilateral nodes
N2	Mobile contralateral or bilateral nodes
N3	Fixed nodes

UICC: International Union Against Cancer.
AJC: American Joint Committee for Cancer Staging.

Table 2 **Sites of primary carcinoma with a high incidence of occult nodes**	
Piriform fossa	Tongue base
Supraglottic larynx	Floor of mouth
Nasopharynx	

patients, prophylactic radiotherapy markedly diminishes the incidence of recurrent neck disease with little increase in morbidity.

N1: Palpable ipsilateral neck nodes

N1 metastatic disease is subclassified into whether the primary site is known or unknown.

N1 with known primary site

In these patients the management of the metastatic neck disease must be considered with the primary tumour. Treatment may be primary radiotherapy or primary surgery, e.g. advanced laryngeal cancer with nodal disease will involve laryngeal surgery and radical neck dissection. However, a squamous carcinoma of the nasopharynx with neck metastases would be treated with radiotherapy.

If primary irradiation fails to control neck disease, a neck dissection is indicated. Neck nodes over 3 cm in diameter are unlikely to be sterilized by radiotherapy and should be primarily treated by surgery. Metastases from thyroid carcinoma are usually managed by local nodal clearance without formal neck dissection.

N1 with no known primary site (occult primary)

The histological appearance of the lymph node may give a clue to where the primary malignant site may be located (Table 3). Metastatic supraclavicular nodes are likely to have been involved from infraclavicular primary malignant sites.

In about a third of cases the occult primary will be uncovered at the time of presentation. Long-term follow-up will unearth malignancy in a further third. However, in a third of cases no primary site is ever discovered (see Fig. 1).

N2: Bilateral neck nodes

The appearance of bilateral malignant metastatic neck nodes is a very poor prognostic sign. Such an event is more likely in primary tumours of the tongue base and hypopharynx. Serious thought should be given as to whether such patients require active treatment or active palliation. It is feasible to perform bilateral neck dissection as a single rather than staged procedure, preserving one jugular vein. Tying a single internal jugular vein results in a rise in intracranial pressure which is even further raised on tying the second side (Fig. 3). Morbidity and mortality

related to the huge increase in intracranial pressure may be prevented by modification of the classic radical dissection.

N3: Fixed nodes

Fixity of nodes is a subjective evaluation. A node may become fixed due to sheer size or if it has burst its capsule and, therefore, surrounding tissue has become invaded with malignant disease. It is a rare event but not necessarily a contraindication to surgical resection. Fixation to skin may be overcome by skin excision and replacement of tissue with local or distant flaps. Invasion of the carotid can be treated by resection and interposition of a vein graft. Fixation to the skull base and brachial plexus indicates that the disease is incurable, and terminal care support is initiated.

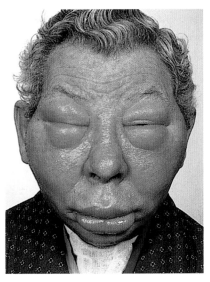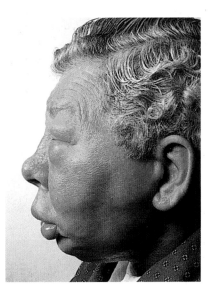

Fig. 3 **Severe oedema of head and neck.** This occurred after tying the internal jugular vein during a radical neck dissection when the other side had been operated on some years previously.

Table 3 The occult primary — how the histology of a malignant node may assist in determining the primary site

Histology of metastatic neck node	Probable primary malignant sites
Squamous cell carcinoma	**Head and neck sites:** nasopharynx, tonsil, tongue base, supraglottic larynx, floor of mouth, piriform fossa, postcricoid region
Adenocarcinoma	**Infraclavicular sites:** bronchus, stomach, breast, intestine, kidney, prostate, uterus
	Head and neck sites: ethmoid sinuses and thyroid gland
Undifferentiated or anaplastic carcinoma	Exclude lymphoma by immunocytochemistry Consider the above sites of carcinoma

Neck lumps — management of malignant lumps

- The commonest cause of a lateral neck swelling is an enlarged lymph node, usually secondary to inflammatory, lymphomatous or metastatic disease.
- The commonest primary sites of malignant neck nodes are metastatic squamous carcinoma from the head and neck.
- Metastatic adenocarcinoma, particularly if the nodes are low in the neck, may be from infraclavicular sites.
- Excisional rather than incisional biopsies of neck nodes should be performed to avoid implanting malignant disease.
- Occult nodes (primary malignant site known) are defined as impalpable nodes. Prophylactic neck radiotherapy should be considered to control the potential neck disease.
- N1 nodes should be treated together with the primary site. If the primary site is unknown (occult primary), a thorough investigation and continued follow-up will reveal it in 60% of cases.
- The standard surgical procedure for treating malignant nodal disease in the neck is a radical neck dissection.

Laryngeal neoplasia

Most cancerous lesions in the larynx should be diagnosed early as their site of localization leads to an immediate alteration in voice. Respiratory symptoms usually develop late.

Benign laryngeal tumours

Benign laryngeal tumours are encountered only infrequently, the most common being the haemangiomata of childhood and respiratory papillomatosis (p. 65).

Benign cartilaginous tumours are also rare and tend to occur in the cricoid cartilage. There is progressive narrowing of the airway, particularly the subglottis, leading to dyspnoea and inspiratory stridor. These chondromas may be apparent clinically and are demonstrated on plain X-rays or CT scan (Fig. 1). Conservative surgery is the treatment of choice, as these benign tumours are extremely slow growing.

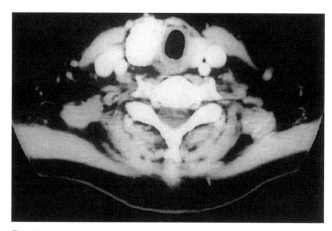

Fig. 1 **A CT scan of a huge cricoid chondroma.**

The granular cell myoblastoma, despite its name, arises from Schwann cells rather than muscle cells. The tumour tends to be localized to the true vocal cords, thereby causing dysphonia. Histologically, it may be mistaken for squamous cell carcinoma. Provided the clinician is aware of this pitfall, the tumour can be treated by simple local endoscopic excision.

Paragangliomas (chemodectomas; glomus tumours) may occur in the larynx and usually present as painful lesions causing dysphagia (Fig. 4, p. 115). The diagnosis is confirmed histologically, and the majority require conservative surgery.

Malignant laryngeal tumours

The majority of malignant laryngeal cancers are squamous cell carcinomas. Adenocarcinoma, adenoid cystic carcinoma, sarcoma and lymphoma are extremely rare.

Verrucous carcinoma of the larynx is a special case. This has macroscopic features of malignancy, but microscopically may appear benign. However, malignant features are seen if the histological examination is thorough and detailed. It is best treated with radiotherapy.

The classification of laryngeal malignant disease is shown in Table 1. For descriptive purposes, the larynx is divided into three regions: the supraglottis, glottis and subglottis. It is useful to discuss the management of malignant laryngeal disease according to the region primarily affected. The common symptoms are illustrated by region in Figure 2.

T1S — carcinoma in situ

T1S is the stage of laryngeal carcinoma that may precede frank invasive malignant disease. Histologically, the carcinoma does not breach the basement membrane. The affected area is excised under microscopic control using either microinstruments or a carbon dioxide laser. Clearly all lesions should be biopsied prior to vaporization with the laser beam.

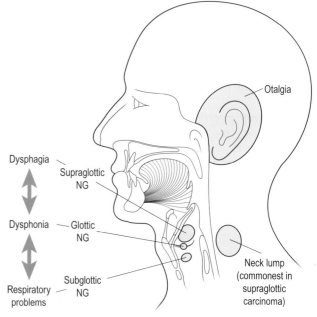

Fig. 2 **Symptoms of laryngeal neoplasia.** The commonest symptom for each region of the larynx is illustrated. Enlargement will result in additional symptoms due to spread to adjacent regions or metastatic disease. (NG: neoplastic growth)

Supraglottic laryngeal carcinoma

The sites of tumour in the supraglottic region (Fig. 2) include the lower portion of the epiglottis, false cords, ventricles and arytenoids. A very rich decussating lymphatic supply is present, so the frequency of regional nodal metastases is high and may be bilateral.

Clinical features

Malignancy in the supraglottis presents late due to the potential space available for expansion. Voice changes tend

Table 1 **Classification of the primary site of carcinoma of the larynx**	
Designation	**Description**
T1S	Carcinoma in situ
T1	Carcinoma within one region
T2	Carcinoma in 2 regions but with mobile vocal cords
T3	Fixation of vocal cord
T4	Carcinoma beyond the larynx (e.g. thyroid, tongue, hypopharynx)

The nodal (N) and distant metastasis (M) status will allow formal TNM classification.

to be late features. The patient may present with dysphagia, respiratory problems or with a metastatic neck node.

Modern MRI or CT scanning provides excellent images for assessing the extent of the neoplasia (Fig. 4). Endoscopic laryngoscopy allows a full assessment of the extent of the disease, and the precise nature of the disease is confirmed by biopsy. The neck should be painstakingly palpated to detect the presence of any metastatic neck nodes.

Management
Treatment in a few highly selected cases (patients with no neck disease, no spread to adjacent regions and fully mobile cords) may be supraglottic laryngectomy. This form of partial laryngectomy resects the diseased area but allows voice retention. Postoperatively, there is often some aspiration of food and drink. This aspiration may be so severe and persistent that total laryngectomy with an end tracheostome may be required.

For the majority of patients, radiotherapy to the primary site and neck nodes is recommended, with assiduous follow-up. Total laryngectomy and radical neck dissection is reserved for residual or recurrent disease.

Glottic laryngeal carcinoma
Glottic laryngeal carcinoma is the most common malignant tumour of the larynx. It usually commences on the free vibrating edge of the true vocal cord and can spread in any direction (Fig. 3). Anterior spread to the anterior commissure is a poor prognostic sign as this site is close to cartilage and allows further easy spread to the thyroid gland. Lateral spread into muscle will impair the mobility of the cords and may also reach lymphatic channels. The true cord is devoid of

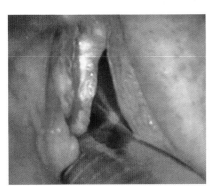

Fig. 3 **Squamous carcinoma of the left vocal cord.**

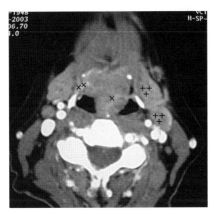

Fig. 4 **Axial CT scan of a supraglottic carcinoma (x). Note erosion of thyroid cartilage (xx) and neck node metastasis (⁺₊⁺).**

any lymphatic supply and, hence, lesions confined just to the cord have an excellent prognosis.

Clinical features
The earliest symptom of glottic cancer is dysphonia (hoarseness). Any patient with dysphonia persisting for 4 weeks should be seen by an ENT surgeon to have the larynx formally assessed. Other symptoms appear late in the disease process due to spread beyond the glottis or to extralaryngeal structures (Fig. 2).

Management
Radiotherapy is advocated for virtually all glottic tumours. T1 lesions will have over a 95% cure rate with this modality. Virtually all other stages should be treated similarly, with the neck being irradiated in those with nodal disease. Primary surgery may be necessary in patients who present with advanced disease.

Total laryngectomy with a radical neck dissection may be required in cases of residual or recurrent disease. Partial laryngectomy may be feasible in a small group of patients, allowing them to retain a functional voice (p. 100).

Subglottic laryngeal carcinoma
The subglottis is the least frequent site of laryngeal carcinoma. It is a region of rich lymphatics that drain to the paratracheal and cervical regional nodes. Subglottic carcinoma has a propensity to spread inferiorly into the trachea and anteriorly into the thyroid gland.

Clinical features
Dysphonia occurs if the spread of disease extends superiorly to involve the glottis. Generally, dysphonia is a late feature with the patient more

likely to present in respiratory distress or even obstruction. The role of tracheostomy is controversial in such instances as some clinicians would advocate an urgent total laryngectomy.

Management
The management of subglottic carcinoma without evidence of metastatic nodal disease is with radiotherapy and regular post-treatment endoscopic reviews to detect recurrent disease. Surgery is the preferred choice in patients with nodal disease, or for residual or recurrent disease after radiotherapy.

Transglottic laryngeal carcinoma
Malignant squamous tumours can involve all three regions of the larynx at time of presentation. Most have a period of symptomatic growth. Presentation is usually with onset of respiratory obstruction or the appearance of neck nodes.

Emergency tracheostomy may be required due to respiratory difficulties. Radiotherapy is the preferred treatment in patients without regional nodal disease.

In the presence of neck disease, laryngectomy with radical neck dissection is the primary form of treatment. However, some clinicians regard primary radiotherapy to larynx and neck as the correct first step in management, with surgery reserved to salvage residual or recurrent disease.

Laryngeal neoplasia

- The majority of laryngeal lesions are malignant.

- 60% occur in the glottis and present early due to the onset of dysphonia.

- Dysphonia is usually a late presentation symptom of subglottic and supraglottic malignancy.

- A supraglottic carcinoma may present as a metastatic neck lump.

- T1S (carcinoma in situ) should be treated by regular stripping of the vocal cord or laser cordectomy, with histological review.

- Radiotherapy is the primary form of treatment in laryngeal carcinoma without evidence of nodal disease.

- Primary surgery to the larynx and neck may be advocated for patients with evidence of metastatic neck disease. Surgery is most commonly reserved for residual or recurrent disease after primary radiotherapy.

Laryngeal surgery and post-laryngectomy rehabilitation

Any operation on the larynx has the potential to compromise the local functions of respiration, speech and swallowing. The degree to which each physiological function is undermined depends on the precise operation and the success of postoperative rehabilitation.

There are essentially two types of procedures for laryngeal cancer: partial or total laryngectomy.

Partial laryngectomy

Partial laryngectomy is only infrequently performed in the UK, as most amenable lesions have excellent cure rates with primary radiotherapy. More recently the endoscopic use of carbon dioxide laser has given good results for laryngeal carcinomas that previously may have been suitable for partial laryngectomy.

In general the selection of patients for such procedures is very strict, and the majority of laryngeal carcinomas do not fulfill the necessary criteria.

Total laryngectomy

Total laryngectomy is most frequently indicated for residual or recurrent laryngeal cancer, after failure of primary radiotherapy. Rarer indications include a functionally useless larynx secondary to laryngeal trauma, particularly if voice quality is poor and there is a life-threatening risk of aspiration of food and drink.

In total laryngectomy part of the pharynx is included in the resection and the cut end of the trachea is relocated in the skin of the anterior neck as an end tracheostome. The defect in the pharynx is closed with sutures over a temporary nasogastric feeding tube and generally heals within 10–14 days.

Complications of total laryngectomy

The main problems associated with total laryngectomy are shown in Table 1.

Pharyngocutaneous fistulae

Pharyngocutaneous fistulae are tracts connecting the pharynx to the skin of the neck. They may be multiple and leak saliva (Fig. 1). There is an increased risk of developing such fistulae if the surgical technique is

Table 1 **Complications after total laryngectomy**
Voice loss
Pharyngocutaneous fistulae
Tracheal crusting
Stomal recurrence
Dysphagia
Thyroid and parathyroid defects

poor, preoperative radiotherapy has been given and the patient is poorly nourished. The majority of fistulae will heal spontaneously over a period of weeks. However, those associated with loss of tissue will require repair with skin flaps.

Tracheal crusting

Tracheal crusting is not uncommon. It is prevented by regular tracheal suction, constant humidification of inspired air and adequate environmental temperature control. It tends to resolve spontaneously after several days.

Hypothyroidism

Hypothyroidism will only occur if the whole thyroid gland is included in the laryngectomy specimen. Nevertheless, thyroid insufficiency may gradually supervene over a period of several years, even if one thyroid lobe remains in situ.

Parathyroid gland insufficiency

Parathyroid gland insufficiency is most likely if a total thyroidectomy is performed. Hypoparathyroidism may occur insidiously.

Dysphagia

Dysphagia is invariable in the first few postoperative days and is due to the

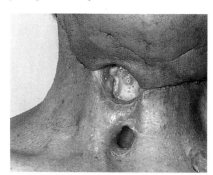

Fig. 1 **Pharyngocutaneous fistulae.** The inferiorly placed hole is an end tracheostome after laryngectomy. The superior defect is a pharyngocutaneous fistula: note the evidence of saliva accumulating in the defect.

presence of the feeding nasogastric tube, and pain. Late dysphagia, developing months or years after surgery, is frequently due to a fibrous stricture at the site of the pharyngeal repair. This will require dilatation.

Recurrence of disease

Recurrence of disease in the end tracheostome has a poor prognosis (Fig. 2). It may be due to implantation of tumour cells during the primary laryngectomy, or a new primary cancer at the stomal site. The majority of such patients will be managed as terminal cases. Palliative radiotherapy and surgery may alleviate the distressing symptoms of respiratory distress and fungating skin mass.

Voice restoration after laryngectomy

Serious psychological stress and loss of self-esteem may develop in the laryngectomy patient. It is essential therefore to enlist the assistance of a speech therapist to help in preoperative counselling and postoperative rehabilitation.

Voice restoration after total laryngectomy can be effected by producing a phonatory sound either by using the oesophagus, or with an external source of sound (artificial larynx).

Oesophageal speech

Oesophageal speech is based on a portion of the oesophagus called the pharyngo-oesophageal (PE) segment.

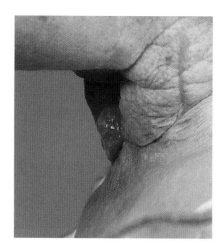

Fig. 2 **An end tracheostome with evidence of florid recurrent carcinoma.**

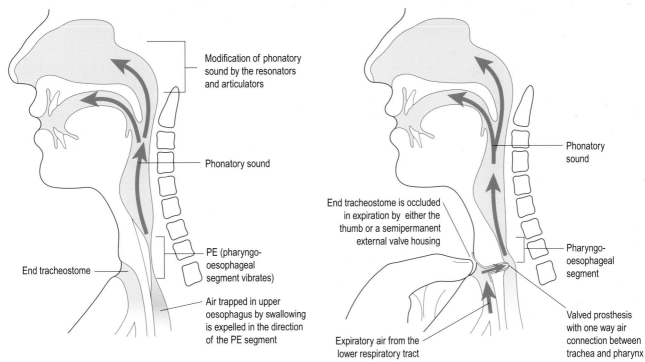

Fig. 3 **The principles of oesophageal speech after total laryngectomy.**

Fig. 4 **The principles of neoglottic speech after total laryngectomy.**

It involves the rapid swallowing of air which is trapped in the upper part of the oesophagus (Fig. 3). This air reservoir is employed to vibrate the PE segment by controlled contraction of the thoracic and abdominal muscles. The phonatory sound produced is modified in the normal way by the resonators and articulatory mechanisms in the oral cavity and nose. In effect, the oesophagus has replaced the lungs as a small power source for initiating vibration. Only about 20% of laryngectomy patients achieve speech in this way. Oesophageal speech can only be acquired with long-term speech therapy and many patients never achieve a satisfactory quality.

Neoglottic speech

Various surgical techniques employ valved prostheses which are inserted to redirect pulmonary air through the PE segment. The prosthesis is placed in a surgically created fistula connecting the posterior tracheal and anterior oesophageal walls (Fig. 4). The one-way valve in the prosthesis allows air to flow into the PE segment when the stoma is occluded during exhalation. More recently, external valve housings have been employed to overcome the tedium and inconvenience of finger occlusion. The major complication of surgical prosthetic techniques is the risk of a leak around the tracheo-

oesophageal valve, allowing aspiration of food, drink and saliva.

Artificial larynx

Artificial larynxes (Fig. 5) work on the principle that air within the vocal tract can be put into vibration by an external battery powered device. The

instrument can be either placed against the skin of the neck or in the oral cavity.

Speech production in this technique sounds very mechanical, and it is difficult to reproduce alterations in pitch or loudness.

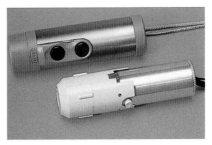
(a)

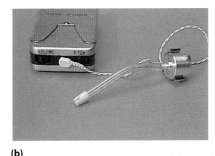
(b)

Fig. 5 **Artificial larynxes. (a)** These are placed externally in the neck to generate vibration in the pharyngo-oesophageal segment. **(b)** An intraoral device: the plastic tube is placed directly into the mouth to generate a phonatory sound.

Laryngeal surgery and rehabilitation

- Total laryngectomy is almost exclusively performed for malignant disease of the larynx.
- In total laryngectomy, part of the pharyngo-oesophagus is included in the resection.
- Voice loss is the severest complication of total laryngectomy.
- Oesophageal speech is produced by expelling air trapped in the upper oesophagus with a satisfactory result in only about 1 in 5 patients.
- Artificial larynxes are easy to use but produce an unnatural, mechanical sound.
- Neoglottic procedures involve the creation of a tracheo-oesophageal connection to utilize pulmonary air to vibrate the PE segment.
- Surgical voice prostheses are easily inserted, but require considerable perseverence to acquire the skills needed to effectively use and care for them.

Neoplasia of the oral cavity

The anatomical contents of the oral cavity are shown in Figure 1. These include the upper and lower alveolus, teeth, lips and the anterior two-thirds of the tongue.

Virtually all oral cavity cancers are of the malignant squamous cell variety. Adenoid cystic carcinoma can arise from minor salivary glands but is rare. The incidence of squamous carcinoma by site within the oral cavity is shown in Figure 2.

Premalignant lesions in the oral cavity include leucoplakia and erythroplakia (p. 88). In virtually all neoplasia of the oral cavity one or more of several aetiological factors are present. Smoking and alcohol abuse are very common. Chronic dental infection, e.g. caries, may result in malignant change, as may lesions seen in tertiary syphilis.

Carcinoma of the lip

Carcinoma of the lip is common in outdoor workers and in regions close to the equator, presumably due to the effects of ultraviolet light. Tobacco smokers show a higher incidence of lip cancer. Historically, smoking a clay pipe was the major cause.

Clinical features

The lower lip, perhaps due to its greater size, is most frequently affected. Dyskeratosis usually manifests as a white patch on the lip, termed 'actinic cheilitis'.

The appearance of a carcinoma of the lip is usually an ulcer (Fig. 3). Included in the differential diagnosis is keratoacanthoma, syphilis and tuberculosis. A biopsy will confirm the diagnosis.

Management

A lip shave and advancement of the vermillion is performed in actinic

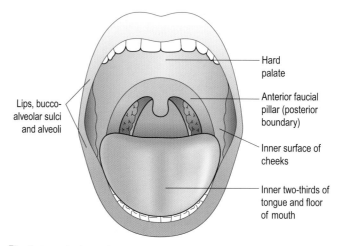

Fig. 1 **Boundaries and structures within the oral cavity.**

Hard palate
Anterior faucial pillar (posterior boundary)
Inner surface of cheeks
Inner two-thirds of tongue and floor of mouth
Lips, bucco-alveolar sulci and alveoli

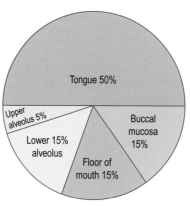

Fig. 2 **The incidence of squamous carcinoma in the oral cavity by site.**

Tongue 50%
Upper alveolus 5%
Lower 15% alveolus
Floor of mouth 15%
Buccal mucosa 15%

cheilitis. Any neoplastic lesion requiring less than a third of the lip to be excised can be removed by a modified V incision and primary closure (Fig. 4). Larger tumours will require local skin flaps for reconstruction. Radical neck dissection will be necessary if metastatic nodal disease is present. Radiotherapy in small early lesions also produces excellent results, and control may be achieved using the argon laser.

Carcinoma of the tongue

The incidence of tongue cancer is diminishing due to improvements in dental hygiene and the fall in popularity of chewing tobacco. The lateral border of the tongue is the commonest site affected.

Clinical features

A persistent ulcer, usually painless, is the common presentation (Fig. 5). If allowed to grow, the lesion will ultimately cause tongue fixation and

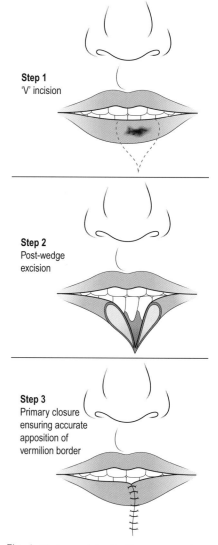

Step 1
'V' incision

Step 2
Post-wedge excision

Step 3
Primary closure ensuring accurate apposition of vermilion border

Fig. 4 **Wedge excision for lip cancer can be employed if less than 30% of lip is involved.**

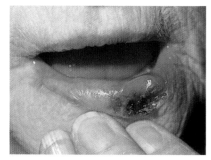

Fig. 3 **A squamous cell carcinoma of the lower lip.**

invade the mandible. The patient will then experience difficulty in chewing, swallowing and speech. About a third of patients will have a metastatic neck

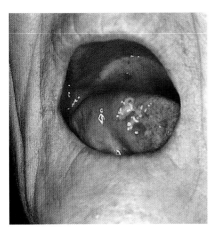

Fig. 5 **A carcinoma of the tongue.**

gland at presentation, which may be on the contralateral side of the neck due to the decussating nature of the lymphatic drainage in this area. The diagnosis is confirmed by biopsy.

Management
Treatment of small lesions without neck metastases is by either surgery or radiotherapy. A wedge excision may be employed, but implanted radium needles can produce the same cure rate. Larger lesions will require a partial glossectomy, resection of the mandible and neck dissection.

Carcinoma of floor of mouth
Squamous carcinoma at this site tends to present late. Most lesions will have already invaded the periosteum and bone of the mandible.

Clinical features
Dysphagia or odynophagia (pain on swallowing) are common symptoms. Pain is usually a major feature and signifies deep invasion. There may also be referred otalgia. An orthopantogram or CT may reveal bone erosion of the mandible (Fig. 6). Biopsy is mandatory for tissue diagnosis and prior to embarking on major surgery.

Management
Radiotherapy is usually not offered as a primary form of treatment as any subsequent excision has a high risk of producing osteoradionecrosis of irradiated bone. After surgical excision, the soft tissue defect is reconstructed using either a pedicled or free flap. Mandibular reconstruction is also feasible. A radical neck dissection will be required as the presence of nodal disease is almost universal.

Carcinoma of the alveolar ridge
The lower alveolar ridge is most commonly affected. In the elderly, an ill-fitting denture may be the presenting symptom. Most lesions will have spread to bone and the adjacent floor of mouth. The mandible is either invaded directly by tumour or via the inferior dental nerve canal. In the latter case the contiguous spread may be as far posteriorly as the skull base.

Treatment is along similar lines to that of carcinoma of the floor of mouth.

Carcinoma of the hard palate
Squamous carcinoma is rare in this site. Adenoid cystic carcinoma is not uncommon, as are benign minor salivary gland tumours. The former cancer tends to extend along the perineural spaces of the greater palatine nerves and may spread into the cranium.

Treatment of adenoid cystic carcinoma is surgery, possibly followed by postoperative radiotherapy. Any defect in the hard palate can be occluded with a dental obturator.

Carcinoma of the buccal lining
The buccal lining is a very common site for cancer on the Indian subcontinent, probably resulting from metaplastic change included by betel nut chewing. The lesion may be ulcerative or exophytic (Fig. 7). A biopsy will confirm the diagnosis. Early small lesions may be successfully excised and primarily sutured. Wider resection will require skin grafting. Radiotherapy should be used in extensive lesions, which are usually incurable due to invasion of the pterygoid muscle region.

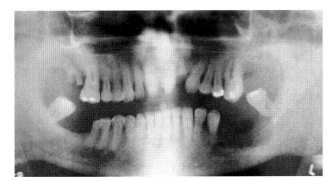

Fig. 6 **An orthopantogram showing erosion of the left mandible due to extension of a carcinoma in the floor of the mouth.**

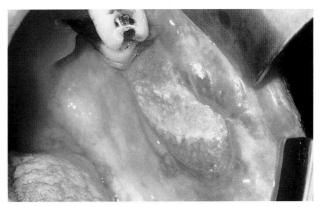

Fig. 7 **An extensive carcinoma of the buccal mucosa.**

Neoplasia of the oral cavity

- The majority of malignant tumours in the oral cavity present as ulcers.
- Syphilis and tuberculosis are now infrequent causes of ulcers in the oral cavity.
- Palpation of a lesion in the oral cavity will yield more information (texture, dimensions, fixity, etc.) than visual inspection.
- Any ulcer in the oral cavity if present for more than 3 weeks must be biopsied to exclude malignant disease.
- Biopsy is mandatory prior to any surgery.
- Osteoradionecrosis may occur in post-irradiated bone if damaged surgically.
- Soft tissue surgical defects are best replaced so as to maintain mobility in any tongue remnant and to aid mastication and articulation.

Neoplasia of the oropharynx

The anatomical dimensions of the oropharynx have been previously detailed (p. 56). The major sites comprising the oropharynx are illustrated in Figure 1. The majority of tumours are malignant squamous cell carcinomas, but lymphoma and minor salivary gland lesions can also occur (Fig. 2). Benign tumours are rarely encountered.

Squamous carcinoma of the oropharynx

Squamous carcinoma of the oropharynx is a disease predominantly of the elderly male, with the tonsil and faucial pillars being the site of incidence in 50% of cases (Fig. 3). Due to the rich lymphatic supply of the oropharynx, the regional lymph nodes are involved in about 60% of cases.

Clinical features

The usual presentation is a history of throat discomfort associated with progressive dysphagia and otalgia. Many patients have a sensation of a 'lump in the back of the throat'. About 40% present with a metastatic neck node. The tumour is usually apparent as an ulcer on routine examination (Fig. 4), but its margins are more clearly determined by palpation and MRI scanning.

A chest X-ray is mandatory, and radiology of the mandible may reveal bony invasion. A full assessment of the extent of the lesion and a biopsy are necessary and may entail a general anaesthetic.

Management

Patients may be incurable due to the presence of bilateral nodes, anaplastic carcinoma or distant metastases. For the remainder, treatment is either surgery or radiotherapy, although combination therapy is frequently employed.

In the absence of metastatic neck nodes, radiotherapy is given as the primary treatment modality, with surgery reserved for failures. In the presence of neck nodes the approach is *com*bined neck dissection, *mandi*bulectomy and resection of the *o*ropharynx – the so called 'commando' operation. A pedicled myocutaneous skin flap or free microvascular graft can be used to reconstruct the tissue defect created (Fig. 5).

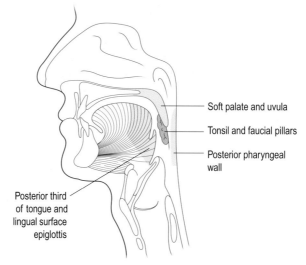

Fig. 1 **The major sites within the oropharynx.**

Soft palate and uvula
Tonsil and faucial pillars
Posterior pharyngeal wall
Posterior third of tongue and lingual surface epiglottis

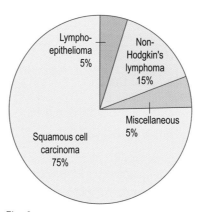

Fig. 2 **The incidence of oropharyngeal neoplasia according to histological type.**

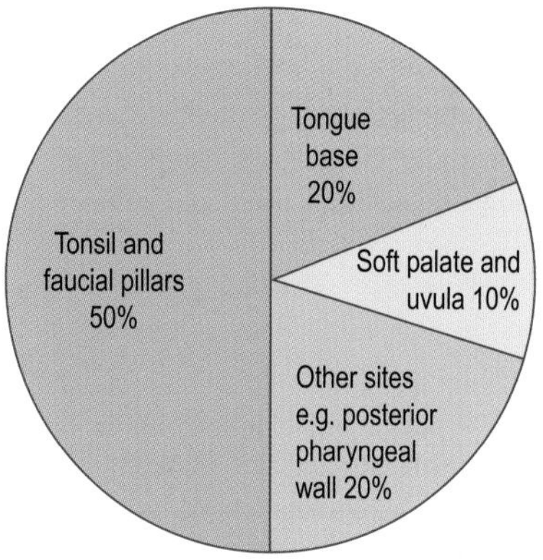

Lympho-epithelioma 5%
Non-Hodgkin's lymphoma 15%
Miscellaneous 5%
Squamous cell carcinoma 75%

Fig. 3 **The site of incidence of squamous cell carcinoma in the oropharynx.**

Tongue base 20%
Soft palate and uvula 10%
Tonsil and faucial pillars 50%
Other sites e.g. posterior pharyngeal wall 20%

Prognosis

The overall survival of patients is dependent on the oropharyngeal site and the size of the carcinoma. The survival from tonsil squamous carcinoma is greater than in lesions of the tongue base. Overall, only 25% of patients survive 5 years.

Lymphoepithelioma of the oropharynx

A variant of squamous carcinoma is the lymphoepithelioma. It shows certain important characteristics. There is a wide presence of lymphocytes in the lesion so that histological confusion with lymphoma may occur. Immunocytochemistry will be required in cases where the squamous cell component is not easily apparent with routine staining techniques.

Lymphoepithelioma is encountered in the tonsil, base of tongue and

nasopharynx. It has a tendency to spread to local and distant sites, but fortunately is extremely radiosensitive.

Lymphoma of the oropharynx

The oropharynx is the commonest extranodal site for lymphomata. These are mostly non-Hodgkin's lymphoma (NHL) of the B-cell variety and of high-grade malignancy. T-cell NHL is much less frequent and usually associated with immunosuppressive disease such as AIDS (p. 86).

Clinical features

The tonsil is the usual site affected and presents as a smooth unilateral enlargement of this structure (Fig. 6). A tonsillectomy will be required, and the specimen examined histologically to determine the cellular immunology and the surface markers. Staging of NHL requires a chest X-ray and CT or MRI of the thorax and abdomen (Fig. 7).

Management

Treatment involves radiotherapy for localized lymphoma, and over two-thirds of patients will be cured. Disseminated NHL is treated by cytotoxic agents. Single agents are employed for low-grade lymphomata and combination chemotherapy for histologically high-grade lymphomata.

Salivary gland tumours of the oropharynx

Salivary gland tumours are rare in the oropharynx. About 50% are due to malignant adenoid cystic carcinoma arising from the tonsil. This neoplasm is extremely aggressive with a propensity to spread along perineural lymphatics and to metastasize to the lung. Benign salivary gland tumours are invariably pleomorphic adenomata.

Management

Treatment is surgical excision for both benign and malignant lesions. Adenoid cystic carcinoma is treated by wide excision radical surgery, reconstructive procedures and postoperative radiotherapy.

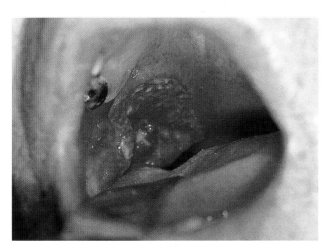

Fig. 4 **An ulcerating carcinoma of the right tonsil.**

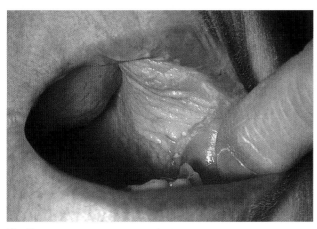

Fig. 5 **A myocutaneous flap inserted into the oropharynx and oral cavity after resection of the primary cancer.**

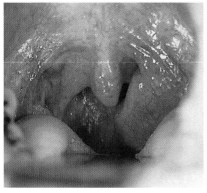

Fig. 6 **Unilateral smooth tonsil swelling due to non-Hodgkin's lymphoma.**

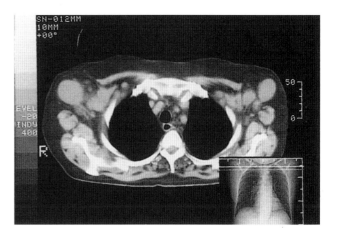

(a)

(b)

Fig. 7 **Whole body CT scan with non-Hodgkin's lymphoma.**
(a) Enlarged axillary nodes. (b) Grossly enlarged spleen and para-aortic nodes.

Neoplasia of the oropharynx

■ Oropharyngeal cancer may present as a 'lump in the back of the throat'.

■ Virtually all oropharyngeal lesions can be visualized on routine examination.

■ All oropharyngeal lesions should be palpated. This allows accurate assessment of the extent of the lesion.

■ A unilateral enlargement of the tonsil requires excision and histological assessment.

■ Squamous cell carcinoma is the commonest neoplastic lesion encountered in the oropharynx.

■ 40% of patients with an oropharyngeal carcinoma present with a metastatic neck node.

■ The tonsil is the commonest site for extranodal lymphomata; the majority of these are of the non-Hodgkin's B-cell variety.

Neoplasia of the hypopharynx

The hypopharynx (laryngopharynx) extends from the hyoid superiorly to the cricoid cartilage inferiorly. It is subdivided into three parts (Fig. 1).

Benign tumours in this region are rare. Virtually all malignant tumours are squamous carcinomas, and the incidence according to site is shown in Figure 2. Neck node metastases are very common from primary sites within the hypopharynx, with the piriform fossa having the highest incidence. Postcricoid tumours may metastasize to the mediastinal and paratracheal group of nodes, as well as nodes in the neck.

Hypopharyngeal carcinoma
Aetiological factors
Tobacco smoke and alcohol have been implicated in hypopharyngeal

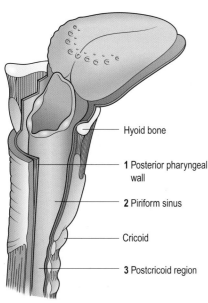

Fig. 1 **A view (from behind) of the three regions within the hypopharynx, with part of the posterior pharyngeal wall removed.**

- Hyoid bone
- **1** Posterior pharyngeal wall
- **2** Piriform sinus
- Cricoid
- **3** Postcricoid region

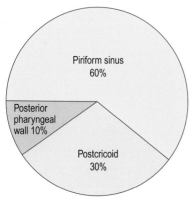

Piriform sinus 60%

Posterior pharyngeal wall 10%

Postcricoid 30%

Fig. 2 **The incidence of squamous cell carcinoma (by region) in the hypopharynx.**

carcinomas. However, despite an increase in tobacco consumption, the incidence of hypopharyngeal cancer does not appear to be rising.

A history of radiation exposure may lead to malignant disease 20–30 years later. This was noted in thyrotoxic patients who were treated by localized radiotherapy to the neck prior to the development of drug therapy.

Paterson–Brown Kelly syndrome
There is a known association between sideropenic dysphagia and postcricoid carcinoma. Paterson and Brown Kelly described a syndrome (also known as Plummer–Vinson) comprising hypochromic microcytic anaemia, glossitis, koilonychia, splenomegaly and a postcricoid web with dysphagia (Fig. 3). It was thought the dysphagia resulted from the presence of the postcricoid web or sometimes a stricture. However, some patients do not demonstrate these obstructive lesions and it is thought likely the dysphagia is due to muscular incoordination.

Haematological abnormalities include a low serum iron and a raised total iron binding capacity. The haemoglobin is frequently low but may be normal. Some patients demonstrate poor

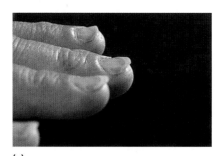

(a)

(b)

Fig. 3 **Paterson–Brown Kelly (Plummer–Vinson) syndrome.** A microcytic anaemia is associated with **(a)** koilonychia, **(b)** glossitis and postcricoid web.

vitamin B_{12} absorption and a low serum vitamin B_{12}. The postcricoid web or a fibrous stricture can be demonstrated radiologically (Fig. 4).

Treatment of sideropenic dysphagia is directed towards correcting the haematological deficits by administration of iron and sometimes vitamin B complex. The dysphagia may resolve, but if it persists, dilatation will be necessary. All cases should be reviewed regularly as a proportion progress to develop postcricoid carcinoma.

Clinical features
The major clinical features of hypopharyngeal neoplasia are summarized in Figure 5. True dysphagia is usually a late feature, as the tumour has considerable space in which to grow prior to causing actual obstructive symptoms. Initially, the only complaint may be odynophagia (pain or discomfort on swallowing) or a feeling of soreness and pricking as food passes through the pharyngo-oesophagus.

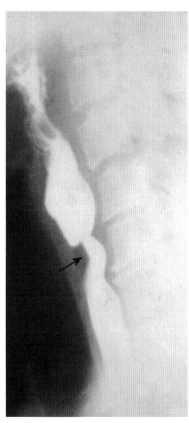

Fig. 4 **A barium swallow illustrating a postcricoid web.**

At the time of presentation, the dysphagia is usually severe and invariably associated with weight loss. Referred otalgia is common. Dysphonia results from either direct invasion of the larynx or vocal cord paralysis caused by involvement of the recurrent laryngeal nerve.

An isolated neck mass due to metastases may be the presenting feature and not accompanied by other symptoms. This is most likely in lesions of the piriform fossa which has a very rich lymphatic supply.

Mirror examination may reveal obvious tumour if it is located in the mouth of the piriform fossa or the posterior pharyngeal wall. Postcricoid lesions lead to pooling of saliva in the hypopharynx. Vocal cord paralysis may also be present.

Investigations

A barium swallow may show an irregular filling defect of the mucosa (Fig. 6). A negative swallow in the presence of persistent feeling of something in the throat requires a formal pharyngo-oesophagoscopy. A chest X-ray may reveal the presence of a second primary cancer or show enlargement of the mediastinum and paratracheal region due to metastatic disease. The lesion should be biopsied and its extent mapped for treatment planning.

Management

Advanced hypopharyngeal tumours can be managed with chemoradiation if there are no neck nodes involved. Surgery can be employed for salvage if this fails or when the primary tumour has neck node metastases.

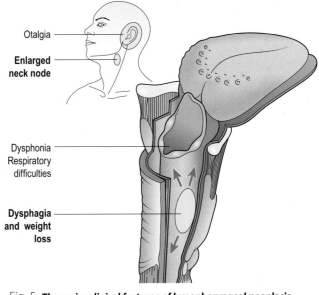

Fig. 5 **The major clinical features of hypopharyngeal neoplasia.**

The standard surgical management for advanced hypopharyngeal tumours involves excision of the larynx and pharynx – total laryngopharyngectomy along with a neck dissection, often bilateral (Fig. 7). Reconstruction of the pharynx and oesophagus involves microvascular free-tissue transfer with a jejunal (small bowel) segment anastomosed to blood vessels in the neck. This type of surgery requires three surgical teams: one to resect the tumour, one to harvest the bowel from the abdomen and one to perform the reconstruction (Fig. 8). This surgery allows the patient to swallow an oral diet.

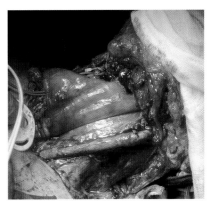

Fig. 8 **Reconstruction with microvascular free jejunal tissue transfer.**

Prognosis

The 5-year survival rates are about 15% with radiotherapy alone, but 30% overall for all forms of treatment.

Neoplasia of the hypopharynx

- Sideropenic dysphagia (Paterson–Brown Kelly or Plummer–Vinson syndrome) is associated with the development of postcricoid carcinoma.

- Hypopharyngeal neoplasia tends to present late.

- The earliest symptom of hypopharyngeal neoplasia may merely be the feeling of something in the throat, e.g. a crumb or hair.

- Dysphagia is usually severe by the time of presentation.

- Regional neck metastases are common.

- All cases will require a barium swallow and endoscopic biopsy.

- Radiotherapy should be reserved for small cancers without nodal metastases.

- A third of patients with hypopharyngeal neoplasia are untreatable.

- Surgical excision usually necessitates a pharyngolaryngo-oesophagectomy.

- The swallowing tube is best reconstructed using some form of visceral interposition.

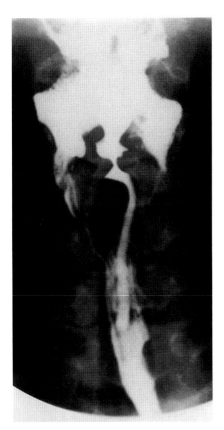

Fig. 6 **A carcinoma of the hypopharynx showing a filling defect on barium swallow.**

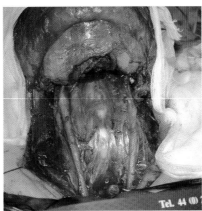

Fig. 7 **Total pharyngolaryngectomy and bilateral neck node dissection for advanced hypopharyngeal cancer.**

Neoplasia of the nasopharynx

The main nasopharyngeal or postnasal space neoplasms are listed in Table 1. Nasopharyngeal carcinoma is the commonest malignant tumour encountered, and the angiofibroma is the only benign tumour of any great importance.

Table 1 **Nasopharyngeal tumours**	
Malignant	**Benign**
Carcinoma	Angiofibroma
Non-Hodgkin's lymphoma	
Chordoma	

Nasopharyngeal carcinoma

The highest incidence of nasopharyngeal carcinoma is in south-east Asia, particularly among patients of Chinese extraction, although other races are affected.

Aetiology

Many factors have been implicated in the development of nasopharyngeal carcinoma. These include ingestion of salted fish, smoke from burning joss sticks, Chinese herbal medicine, cigarette smoking and industrial smoke and chemicals.

The Epstein–Barr virus (EBV) may have a major aetiological role in nasopharyngeal carcinoma. The viral genome appears to become incorporated into nasopharyngeal mucosal cells which may then be triggered by some stimulant to initiate malignant change within the cell.

Clinical features

The majority of tumours arise in the fossa of Rosenmüller and can spread in any direction to produce a vast array of potential symptoms and signs (Fig. 1). A variety of cranial nerve lesions can occur. The involvement of the trigeminal nerve by superior extension into the foramen ovale manifests as facial pain and altered sensation in the face. A Horner's syndrome (meiosis, ptosis and anhidrosis) may result from involvement of the sympathetic trunk in the carotid sheath.

Invasion of the nasopharyngeal end of the Eustachian tube will give rise to otological symptoms such as hearing loss. In any adult Chinese with secretory otitis media it is essential to assume the presence of nasopharyngeal carcinoma until otherwise proven.

Investigations

The neoplasm may be seen on routine postnasal space mirror examination. A more valuable and reliable view will be obtained with the flexible rhinolaryngoscope or rigid nasoendoscope (Fig. 2). It may be feasible to perform a biopsy in outpatients. All other patients should be subjected to formal biopsy under general anaesthesia.

MRI scanning is essential to assess the extent of the disease, particularly its potential extension to the skull base and pharyngeal spaces (Fig. 3). MRI is superior to CT at depicting involvement of soft tissue, but inferior to CT in showing bony destruction.

Epstein–Barr virus antibody titres are useful in assessing the response to treatment, and in detecting subsequent recurrences.

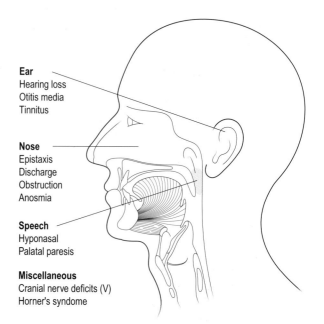

Ear
Hearing loss
Otitis media
Tinnitus

Nose
Epistaxis
Discharge
Obstruction
Anosmia

Speech
Hyponasal
Palatal paresis

Miscellaneous
Cranial nerve deficits (V)
Horner's syndome

Fig. 1 **Clinical features of nasopharyngeal neoplasia.**

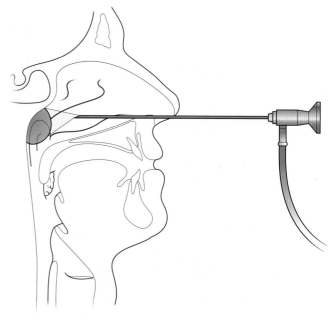

Fig. 2 **Rigid endoscope used to visualize a mass in the nasopharynx.**

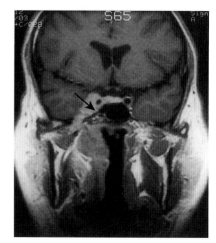

Fig. 3 **MRI scan of a carcinoma of the right nasopharynx.** Note involvement around the internal carotid artery (arrow).

Management

The usual treatment is radiotherapy to both the primary site in the nasopharynx and to the neck, even in the absence of palpable neck nodes. Surgery in the form of radical neck dissection may occasionally be performed. The overall 5-year survival rate is about 35%.

Nasopharyngeal angiofibroma

Although histologically benign, nasopharyngeal angiofibromas are aggressive and spread by local extension. The majority arise at the posterior choanae or nasopharynx, predominantly in young males. The proportion of each element of endothelial vascular or fibrous connective tissue is very variable. Those with a predominant vascular structure are more likely to present with a massive epistaxis.

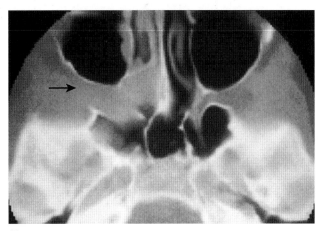

Fig. 4 **A CT scan of a nasopharyngeal angiofibroma.** The arrow shows expansion of the sphenopalatine canal.

Clinical features

Nasal obstruction and epistaxis are the commonest presenting symptoms. However, otological (hearing loss and tinnitus), ocular (diplopia, proptosis) and facial (swelling) symptoms can occur. The mass is readily seen with an indirect mirror, rigid endoscope or flexible rhinolaryngoscope. Biopsy is deferred due to the risk of torrential haemorrhage.

Investigations

Radiological investigations, MRI and CT, will reveal the nature and extent of the angiofibroma (Fig. 4). Angiographic assessment will also allow an opportunity to perform preoperative embolization to reduce the vascularity of the tumour and, hence, minimize blood loss during any subsequent surgical removal (Fig. 5).

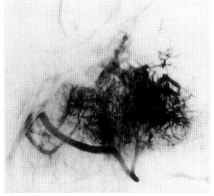 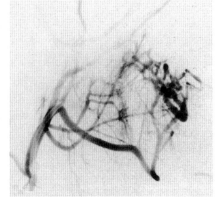

(a)   **(b)**

Fig. 5 **Nasopharyngeal angiofibroma. (a)** Injection of contrast into the maxillary artery shows a very vascular tumour. **(b)** Injection into the same vessel after embolization using particles of polyvinyl alcohol (PVA). The tumour circulation has been ablated.

Management

Radiotherapy should be used only in unresectable lesions as there is a risk of delayed sacromatous change. All other patients require surgical excision, and a variety of approaches, e.g. transpalatal, transantral, lateral rhinotomy or midface degloving, may be needed to adequately remove the angiofibroma.

Other miscellaneous tumours

About 10% of tumours in the nasopharynx are non-Hodgkin's lymphoma. These need to be typed as being either of B- or T-cell origin, and then staged. Cytotoxic therapy with or without radiotherapy is employed to control systemic lymphoma, and radiotherapy is employed alone in localized disease.

The chordoma is a very rare, slow-growing malignant tumour arising from the remnant of the notochord. It can expand from its craniocervical site

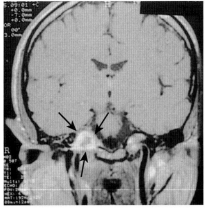

Fig. 6 **MRI scan of chordoma arising in the region of the clivus.**

of origin into the nasopharynx and the neighbouring clivus and cervical vertebrae (Fig. 6). Radical surgical excision or decompression is required as the tumour is not radiosensitive.

Neoplasia of the nasopharynx

- Nasopharyngeal carcinoma is most common in people of Chinese extraction.
- All adults developing secretory otitis media should have their nasopharynx examined by an ENT specialist.
- Nasopharyngeal carcinomas metastasize early and may present as neck nodes.
- Unilateral progressive nasal obstruction and bloody nasal discharge are the earliest symptoms of nasopharyngeal cancer.
- A massive epistaxis in a young adult may be the presenting feature of a nasopharyngeal angiofibroma.
- Adenoidal hypertrophy is *NOT* a cause of nasal obstruction after puberty.
- Radiotherapy is the primary choice of treatment of nasopharyngeal carcinoma.

Neoplasia of the nose and paranasal sinuses

Neoplasia of the nose and paranasal sinuses is rare, occurring in about 1% of all malignancies. Benign tumours are more common than the malignant variety (Table 1).

Table 1 Neoplasms of the nose and paranasal sinuses

Benign	Malignant
Osteoma	Squamous cell carcinoma
Papilloma:	Adenocarcinoma
squamous cell	Transitional cell carcinoma
transitional cell	Olfactory neuroblastoma
	Melanoma

Benign tumours

Squamous papillomata are very common and are located usually in the vestibular skin (Fig. 1). They can be cauterized, but any recurrence should be excised and subjected to histological examination to exclude squamous cell carcinoma.

Transitional cell papillomata (inverted papillomata or Ringertz tumour) usually take origin from the lateral nasal wall. Simple intranasal removal is frequently followed by recurrence. The lesion is more effectively excised by a lateral rhinotomy or midface degloving approach (Fig. 2). About 10% of the benign transitional cell lesions are associated with squamous carcinoma. It is not possible to be sure whether there has been malignant transformation of the benign lesion, or if the carcinoma has occurred de novo.

Benign osteomata are most commonly located in the frontal sinuses and may be first seen as an incidental finding on plain radiology. Symptoms only occur if the frontonasal duct is obstructed. They can grow to an enormous size, although the growth rate is extremely slow. Excision is rarely necessary.

Malignant tumours
Aetiology

Certain factors are known to be carcinogenic in the nose and paranasal sinuses (Table 2). Hardwood dust is a known factor in the development of adenocarcinoma of the ethmoid sinuses. Inhalation of nickel dust is implicated in nasal squamous cell carcinoma. Radiation exposure of the skin of the nose may induce malignant change. About 10% of cases of benign transitional cell papillomata are associated with transitional cell carcinoma.

Clinical features

Clinical features are dependent on the precise location of the malignant tumour. For example, frontal sinus cancer is likely to cause orbital symptoms early in the disease. Nasal cavity lesions may present with nasal obstruction and epistaxis and cause ocular problems only in advanced cases.

Table 2 Aetiological factors implicated in cancer of the nose and sinuses

Nickel dust	Mustard gas
Hardwood dust	Radiation
Transitional cell papilloma	Snuff

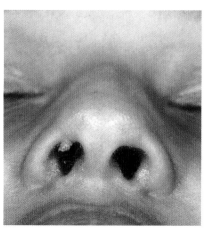
Fig. 1 **A squamous papilloma arising from the nasal vestibule.**

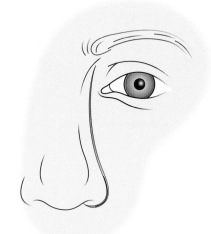
Fig. 2 **The incision for the lateral rhinotomy approach to the nose and paranasal sinuses.**

The majority of malignant disease presents in the maxillary antrum, and this serves to illustrate the major symptoms and signs that may occur (Fig. 3).

Antral tumours usually present late, as the mass must grow to fill the sinus space before causing any major symptoms. Epiphora (watering eye) is due to invasion and blockage of the nasolacrimal duct. A denture which becomes ill fitting is not an uncommon presentation if the lesion grows inferiorly. Facial paraesthesia is due to involvement of the infraorbital nerve in the roof of the antrum, or the trigeminal nerve in the retroantral region. Trismus (reduced jaw opening) is a sign that the pterygoid muscles have been invaded by direct posterior extension.

Investigations

Histological confirmation of the malignant process is usually easy due to the presence of a mass in the nasal cavity. The limits of the disease are most accurately determined by CT

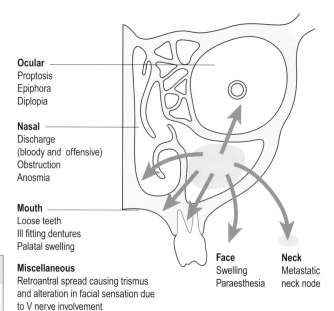

Ocular
Proptosis
Epiphora
Diplopia

Nasal
Discharge
(bloody and offensive)
Obstruction
Anosmia

Mouth
Loose teeth
Ill fitting dentures
Palatal swelling

Miscellaneous
Retroantral spread causing trismus and alteration in facial sensation due to V nerve involvement

Face
Swelling
Paraesthesia

Neck
Metastatic neck node

Fig. 3 **Symptoms and signs in neoplasia of the maxillary antrum.**

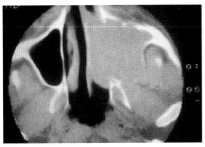

Fig. 4 **A CT scan of carcinoma of the maxillary antrum.** The lesion has extended medially into the nasal cavity, anteriorly into the cheek and posteriorly into the retroantral region.

scanning which can be performed in the coronal and axial planes, and provides useful information about soft tissue invasion (Fig. 4).

Management

The management of malignant disease of the nose and paranasal sinuses is dependent on the histology and the extent of the neoplasm. The majority of cases require full-dose radiotherapy with subsequent planned surgery. The use of systemic and local chemotherapy has been dissapointing. Palliative therapy is extremely valuable, as without some form of treatment the disease is slowly progressive and cosmetically mutilating.

Most malignant disease in the nose and paranasal sinuses may be resected via the lateral rhinotomy approach or by performing a maxillectomy. Any superior extension of the disease into the region of the cribriform plate may be included in the resection by performing a craniofacial resection, i.e. by a combined approach from below and via a craniotomy from above (Fig. 5). If the eye is involved, an orbital exenteration will be necessary.

Prognosis

The overall 5-year survival rate for malignant disease is about 30%. Management is difficult due to late presentation, complex anatomy and the proximity of important structures such as the orbit and cranial contents. CT scanning has proved to be extremely valuable in assessing the extent of the disease, thus resulting in greatly improved management policy.

Non-specific (non-healing midline) granulomata

Non-specific granulomata of the nose and pranasal sinuses are lesions which appear to have clinical features of malignancy but are not true neoplasms. Granulomatous lesions of the nose are frequently due to specific infection, e.g. syphilis, tuberculosis or leprosy. However, the non-specific or non-healing midline granulomata have an unknown aetiology, but have now been classified on histological and clinical grounds (Table 3) into two varieties:

- Wegener's granulomatosis
- lethal midline granuloma (midfacial lymphoma).

Wegener's granulomatosis

Wegener's granulomatosis is a systematic vasculitis of unknown origin. It involves the respiratory tract and kidneys. The nose may be obstructed due to thickened mucosa and crusting. The patient is very unwell, despite the minimal nasal signs. Nasal biopsy may be unhelpful. The diagnosis is made by the presence of granulomata on chest X-ray, abnormal renal function and possibly a positive antineutrophil cytoplasmic antibody test (ANCA). Death occurs usually secondary to kidney failure. High-dose steroids improve renal function and relapses may be prevented with cytotoxic therapy such as cyclophosphamide. Renal transplant can be considered if treatment is successful.

Lethal midline granuloma (midfacial lymphoma)

Lethal midline granuloma is a T-cell lymphoma that results in a slow, progressive destruction of the nose and midface (Fig. 6). Treatment involves a curative dose of radiotherapy, combined with surgical excision of necrotic tissue.

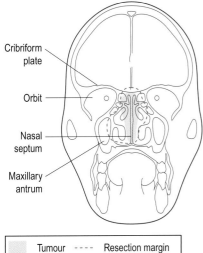

Cribriform plate

Orbit

Nasal septum

Maxillary antrum

| Tumour | - - - - Resection margin |

Fig. 5 **Craniofacial resection.** The area of resection includes the cribriform plate. The orbit and maxilla may be included in the resection.

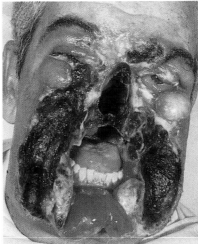

Fig. 6 **Lethal midline granuloma.**

> ### Neoplasia of the nose and paranasal sinuses
>
> - Unilateral nasal obstruction may be due to tumour, nasal polyps or a deflected septum.
> - A bleeding nasal polyp should be biopsied.
> - Neoplasms of the nose and sinuses tend to present late due to the available space for growth.
> - Symptoms and signs may be predominantly nasal, dental, orbital, facial or retroantral depending on the site and direction of spread of malignant disease.
> - The extent of malignant disease is evaluated by CT scanning but MRI may supersede it.
> - The majority of malignant neoplasms will be managed by radiotherapy followed by planned surgery.
> - Extension of disease into the cribriform plate and anterior cranial fossa can be resected by using a cranial approach in combination with the facial route (cf. craniofacial resection).
> - Wegener's granulomatosis is a systemic disease with both the upper and lower respiratory tract and kidney involved.
> - Lethal midline granuloma is a T-cell lymphoma of the nose and midface and is treated with radiotherapy.

Table 3 **The main features of the two types of non-specific, non-healing granulomata of the nose and paranasal sinuses**

Disease	Histological	Clinical	Management
Wegener's granulomatosis	Necrotizing granulomata	Systemic disease	Steroids and cytotoxics
Lethal midline granuloma	T-cell lymphoma	Usually localized to a single site	Radiotherapy

Neoplasia of the salivary glands

The parotid gland accounts for about 80% of cases of salivary gland tumours. The submandibular, sublingual and minor salivary glands comprise the remainder. The majority of parotid tumours are benign, but the incidence of malignancy is high at the other sites.

Salivary gland neoplasia can be divided, depending on the degree of malignancy, into three varieties which are summarized in Table 1 and discussed below. Rare salivary gland neoplasms include lymphoma, haemangioma and metastatic disease.

Table 1 **Classification of salivary gland tumours according to behaviour**	
Classification	**Tumour**
Benign tumours	Benign pleomorphic adenoma
	Monomorphic adenoma (adenolymphoma; Warthin's tumour)
Tumours of variable malignancy	Mucoepidermoid tumour
	Acinic cell tumour
Malignant tumours	Adenoid cystic carcinoma
	Malignant pleomorphic adenoma
	Adenocarcinoma
	Squamous cell carcinoma
	Non-Hodgkin's lymphoma

Benign salivary tumours

Benign pleomorphic adenoma

Virtually all benign pleomorphic adenomas occur in the parotid, with a small number arising in the submandibular gland. The patient usually complains of a painless, slowly enlarging lump in the retromandibular region (Fig. 1). The presence of facial pain or paralysis is indicative of a malignant neoplasm. Pleomorphic adenomas have a false capsule, so that simple enucleation is liable to leave residual tumour. About 10% of these adenomas show malignant tendencies, particularly if left for many years.

Treatment is by parotidectomy. This usually entails resecting the parotid tissue (in which the adenoma is located) superficial to the facial nerve (Fig. 2). Rarely, the tumour may arise in the deep lobe of the parotid and present as an intraoral swelling due to expansion within the parapharyngeal space. In such cases a total parotidectomy with preservation of the facial nerve is performed. A margin of normal tissue should always be excised to ensure that all tumour projections from the main tumour mass are included in the resection.

Warthin's tumour (adenolymphoma)

Warthin's tumour is almost exclusively a disease of the elderly male and is frequently bilateral. It occurs only in the parotid. It presents as an ovoid, mobile, fluctuant mass, usually in the tail of the gland. Painful enlargement may occur in association with upper respiratory tract infections, due to inflammation of the lymphoid tissue contained within the tumour.

Treatment is by surgical excision via a parotidectomy type incision.

Salivary gland tumours of variable malignancy

Mucoepidermoid tumour

Over 90% of mucoepidermoid tumours occur in the parotid gland. If arising from minor salivary glands, the palate is the commonest site. This is the most frequently encountered salivary gland tumour in childhood.

The histological structure determines the behaviour of the tumour. Well-differentiated lesions behave as benign tumours, but an undifferentiated appearance is indicative of a high degree of malignancy with a propensity to local and systemic metastases. Intermediate degrees of malignancy are also encountered.

The histological pattern is only confirmed after parotidectomy. If the facial nerve is involved by disease it should be sacrificed. Postoperative radiotherapy is employed in all cases.

Acinic cell tumour

The acinic cell tumour predominantly arises in the parotid gland. It is extremely slow growing, but about 10% of cases give rise to metastases and a very small number of cases are bilateral. Treatment is by surgical excision with preservation of the facial nerve if it is free of tumour.

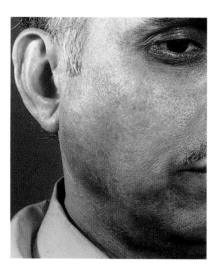

Fig. 1 **A benign pleomorphic adenoma of the right parotid gland.**

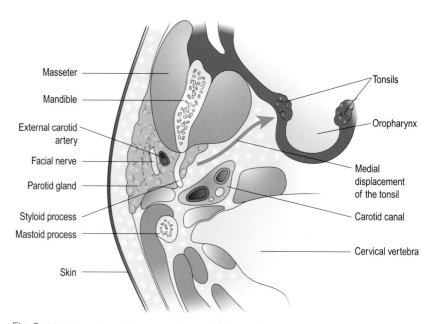

Fig. 2 **Principles of parotid surgery.** A superficial parotidectomy removes all parotid gland tissue superficial to the facial nerve. The deep lobe of the parotid is located deep to the facial nerve; any mass lesion in this region will tend to expand towards the oropharynx causing medial displacement of the tonsil, as shown by the bold arrow.

Masseter
Mandible
External carotid artery
Facial nerve
Parotid gland
Styloid process
Mastoid process
Skin
Tonsils
Oropharynx
Medial displacement of the tonsil
Carotid canal
Cervical vertebra

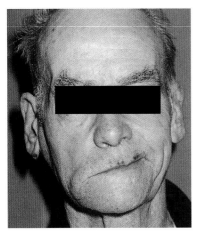

Fig. 3 **An adenoid cystic carcinoma of the parotid with involvement of the facial nerve.**

Malignant salivary gland tumours
Adenoid cystic carcinoma
Adenoid cystic carcinoma is the commonest of the malignant salivary gland neoplasms and tends to be sited in the submandibular, sublingual and minor salivary glands. The parotid is rarely affected.

The presenting feature is usually a swelling, often with pain of several months duration. Latterly, a neck mass may develop. The facial nerve is invariably compromised in tumours arising in the parotid (Fig. 3). The nerve involvement is probably due to the spread of cancer by perineural lymphatics, which is a feature of adenoid cystic carcinoma. Local metastases to lymph nodes are not infrequent. Distant metastases in the lung are also not uncommon.

Treatment is by wide local excision, e.g. excision of the hard palate or total parotidectomy. The facial nerve is sacrificed so as to include cancer cells that will have spread in perineural lymphatics. Grafting the facial nerve is possible by using the sural nerve. A cross-face anastomosis may be offered once the patient is deemed free of tumour. These tumours are radiosensitive, but are rarely cured, with recurrences up to 10 years after treatment. The overall 5-year survival rate is about 60%.

Miscellaneous malignant salivary gland tumours
Adenocarcinoma and squamous cell carcinoma are rare tumours in salivary glands. The prognosis is very poor and wide excision and postoperative radiotherapy are required.

The de novo malignant pleomorphic adenoma of the parotid is extremely rare. The majority arise in a previous, long-existing benign pleomorphic adenoma. The appearance of facial pain or weakness indicates malignant transformation. Radical local surgery, frequently with sacrifice of the facial nerve, and postoperative radiotherapy offer the best hope of cure.

The commonest type of lymphoma of the salivary glands is the non-Hodgkin's variety. A pre-existing Sjögren's syndrome predisposes to the development of lymphoma. After the lymphoma has been staged, treatment is by radiotherapy and/or chemotherapy.

Complications of salivary gland surgery
The major complications of salivary gland surgery are listed in Table 2.

Facial weakness
In parotidectomy, with an intact facial nerve, any facial weakness is usually temporary. It is related to pressure and trauma in the vicinity of the facial nerve. Coagulation diathermy may result in heat damage to the neural elements.

Facial weakness after submandibular gland surgery is due to damage of the mandibular branch of the facial nerve. It rarely recovers.

Anaesthesia of the ear
The great auricular nerve is almost always divided in parotidectomy and results in anaesthesia in the inferior half of the pinna and surrounding skin. The area of anaesthesia may diminish with time, but there is always some residual deficit, particularly of the lobule.

Salivary fistula
A salivary fistula is due to the overproduction of saliva from remaining parotid tissue. It invariably settles spontaneously with pressure dressings and suction drainage.

Table 2 **Complications of salivary gland surgery**	
Procedure	**Complications**
Parotid gland surgery	Facial weakness
	Anaesthesia of ear
	Salivary fistula
	Frey's syndrome (gustatory sweating)
Submandibular gland surgery	Facial weakness
	Tongue weakness
	Anaesthesia of tongue

Frey's syndrome
Frey's syndrome or gustatory sweating is a result of severed parasympathetic fibres destined for the parotid gland rerouting into the skin. Thus, at meal times, the patient experiences pain, inflammation and sweating of the skin over the parotid region. If the symptoms do not settle spontaneously after 6 months, a tympanic nerve section to divide the secretory parasympathetic fibres as they traverse the middle ear may be beneficial.

Weakness and anaesthesia of the tongue
Weakness and anaesthesia of the tongue is due to trauma to the hypoglossal and lingual nerves, respectively, during submandibular gland excision. These complications are permanent (Fig. 4).

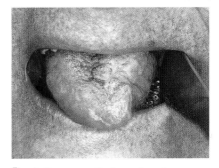

Fig. 4 **Damage to the hypoglossal nerve causes atrophy of the ipsilateral tongue.**

Neoplasia of the salivary glands

- Benign salivary gland tumours usually present as a slowly enlarging, painless mass.
- Facial pain or weakness is invariably due to a malignant salivary tumour.
- Parotidectomy will cure most parotid tumours, as they are benign.
- Malignant salivary gland tumours are more likely to occur in the submandibular and minor salivary glands.
- The facial nerve should be sacrificed if involved by a malignant neoplasm. Immediate nerve grafting or later cross-face anastomosis may be appropriate to overcome the inevitable cosmetic deficit.
- CT and MRI scanning are invaluable in assessing the extent of malignant salivary gland disease, particularly in the parotid and submandibular gland.
- All patients undergoing parotid and submandibular gland surgery should be informed of the risk of permanent facial weakness.

Neoplasia of the ear

Chronic inflammation is a predisposing factor in neoplasia of the ear. Malignant disease in the middle ear is nearly always associated with a history of otorrhoea stretching over several years. Long-term otitis externa may induce cancer in the skin of the ear canal. Exposure to sunlight in pale-skinned individuals has been implicated in the development of basal and squamous cell carcinoma, particularly of the auricle.

Neoplasia of the auricle

The commonest tumours encountered in the auricle are squamous cell and basal cell carcinomas. Rare lesions include malignant melanoma and keratoacanthoma.

Clinical features

The neoplasm usually presents as a slowly progressive ulcer or a persistent area of crusting (Fig. 1). In many cases the lesions may have been present for several years. Lymph node metastases are rarely encountered.

Management

If confined to the outer part of the auricle, the tumour is usually treated by wedge excision and primary suturing. This gives a better cosmetic result and is preferable to radiotherapy. Occasionally, a total auriclectomy is necessary. Nodal disease necessitates a radical neck dissection and such cases should be given postoperative radiotherapy.

Neoplasia of the ear canal

Neoplasms of the ear canal are rare. Those arising in the cartilaginous outer portion of the ear canal offer little resistance to the spread of cancer to the parotid gland and postauricular region (Fig. 2). The deeper bony external canal is a more effective barrier to spread, but the cancer may grow medially into the middle ear. Benign growths in the external ear canal are rarely seen.

Squamous cell carcinoma

The commonest tumour is squamous cell carcinoma. It presents with symptoms of otorrhoea, perhaps tinged with blood, and hearing loss. Facial paralysis occurs if the middle ear is invaded and the facial nerve compromised. Otalgia is

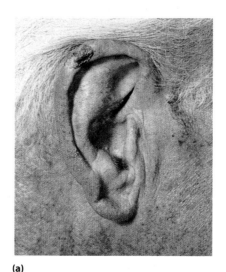
(a)

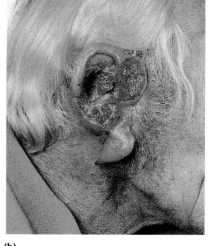
(b)

Fig. 1 **Tumours of the auricle may present either as ulcers or crusts. (a)** A crusting lesion due to a basal cell carcinoma. **(b)** An ulcerating lesion due to squamous carcinoma.

present and increases with the progression of invasion. Squamous cell carcinoma is treated by mastoidectomy and removal of the parotid gland and temporomandibular joint. Postoperative radiotherapy should be given.

Ceruminomas

The term ceruminomas covers all benign and malignant tumours arising from ceruminous glands of the external meatus. (Tumours of the apocrine sweat glands are incorrectly termed as ceruminomas.) Adenoid cystic carcinoma is the most common type of ceruminoma. Radical wide excision surgery is required with postoperative radiotherapy. The prognosis is poor, with the patient dying from local and systemic metastases.

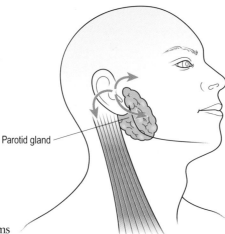
Parotid gland

Fig. 2 **Cancer of the external auditory meatus.** The lesion may spread to the parotid, pre- and postauricular lymph nodes and medially to involve the middle ear.

Neoplasia of the middle ear

Tumours confined purely to the middle ear are rarely encountered. By the time of presentation most will have spread to the external meatus and so it may be difficult to ascertain the primary site of origin. The majority of patients will have a long history of chronic suppurative otitis media with otorrhoea.

Squamous cell carcinoma is the most commonly encountered neoplasm in the middle ear. It spreads by invading bone and will eventually involve the facial nerve, the temporomandibular joint, labyrinth and Eustachian tube. It can spread into the middle cranial fossa and along the skull base to involve the lower cranial nerves as they exit the skull.

Clinical features

The clinical features are illustrated in Table 1. The cardinal feature is the change in the symptom complex of what for several years was a simple discharging ear.

Table 1 **Features of carcinoma of the middle ear**	
Duration of onset	**Clinical feature**
Years	Mucopurulent otorrhoea
Weeks	Bloody otorrhoea
	Progressive otalgia
	Facial paralysis

Investigations

The diagnosis is confirmed by biopsy of aural granulations and polyps. The extent of the disease is determined most suitably with CT scans (Fig. 3) and MRI.

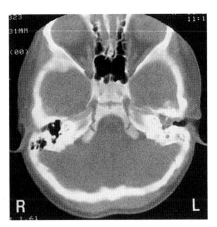

Fig. 3 **A CT scan showing a carcinoma of the left middle ear.**

Management

Some patients may be untreatable because of systemic metastases or poor general health. The most favoured form of treatment is primary surgery and postoperative radiotherapy. The surgery may involve a radical mastoidectomy at the very least, and removal of the temporal bone (petrosectomy) for more extensive disease. The complication rate of the latter procedure is high and includes cerebrospinal fluid leak, meningitis, facial paralysis and damage to the lower cranial nerves. The overall 5-year survival rate is in the order of 30% with combined therapy.

Glomus tumours of the ear

Glomus tumours of the ear arise from the paraganglionic cells (glomus bodies) located at various sites (Fig. 4). The glomus tympanicum arises from the region of the promontory in the middle ear and may present as a middle ear polyp. The glomus jugulare tends to invade the middle ear by bony

erosion and may spread along the skull base to involve the lower cranial nerve (glossopharyngeal, vagus, accessory and hypoglossal). The facial nerve is usually the first and most frequently involved nerve. Intracranial spread is not uncommon as the neoplasm expands.

Clinical features

The commonest symptoms (Table 2) are hearing loss and pulsatile tinnitus. As these features are only slowly progressive, the patient may delay consultation for many years until one of the more distressing late symptoms such as pain appear. Otoscopic examination will reveal either an obvious middle ear polyp, or, if the eardrum is intact, a red or blue swelling behind it (Fig. 5). Biopsy may lead to extensive haemorrhage.

Investigations

The extent of the disease is evaluated by CT and MRI scanning, and this will differentiate between a glomus tympanicum and glomus jugulare (Fig. 6). Angiography is useful in demonstrating the blood supply of the tumour preoperatively.

Management

A glomus tympanicum can usually be resected via a tympanotomy and mastoidectomy approach. The glomus jugulare may be excised after transposing the facial nerve, but can be unresectable due to widespread disease or the patient's general condition. In some cases, radiotherapy is the obvious option as it can reduce both the size and vascularity of the slow-growing tumour and may be effective for several years.

Table 2 **Symptoms of glomus tumours**
Hearing loss *
Pulsatile tinnitus *
Otorrhoea (bloody)
Vertigo
Cranial nerve deficits

*Commonest features.

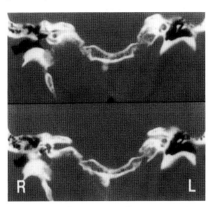

Fig. 5 **The otoscopic appearance of a glomus tympanicum.**

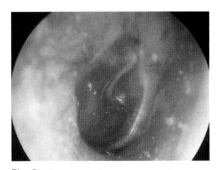

Fig. 6 **A CT scan of a glomus jugulare with bony erosion of the right skull base.**

Neoplasia of the ear

- The majority of auricular tumours can be treated by wedge excision and primary repair.
- Ceruminoma is a misnomer. This is a collective term for both benign and malignant tumours arising from apocrine sweat glands.
- Carcinoma of the middle ear and mastoid tends to arise in a pre-existing and active chronic suppurative otitis media.
- Any changes in the character of chronic otorrhoea or the appearance of otalgia, unsteadiness or facial weakness may be due to malignant transformation in the middle ear.
- CT and MRI scanning are essential in the assessment of both middle ear carcinoma and glomus tumours.
- Temporal bone resection for middle ear carcinoma has a high morbidity.
- A pulsatile tinnitus and hearing loss are the commonest symptoms of glomus tympanicum and jugulare.
- Biopsy of a glomus tumour may result in torrential haemorrhage.
- Radiotherapy may temporarily arrest or considerably slow the growth of glomus tumours.

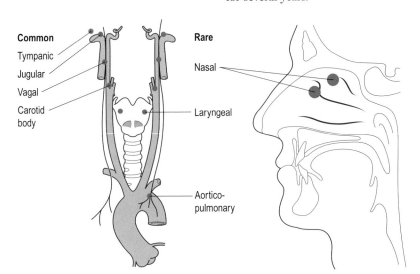

Fig. 4 **Sites of glomus bodies which may give rise to glomus body tumours.**

Terminal care

Malignant disease of the head and neck may be considered to be incurable at the time of presentation, or after medical and surgical treatment. As the disease progresses, severe physical and psychological handicaps are often encountered. At this point in the clinical management it is vital to inform the patient and the close relatives precisely of the gravity and eventual outcome of the disease.

Such patients require specialized care in the management of their terminal cancer. In modern clinical practice this usually involves a 'terminal care' support team comprising hospital-based clinicians and nursing staff, but also community-based paramedics specializing in caring for the dying.

Management principles

The management of terminal head and neck cancer requires control of symptoms, and moral and psychological support to cope with the prospect of dying (Table 1).

Table 1 Major symptoms to be controlled in terminal head and neck neoplasia
Chronic pain
Respiratory difficulties
Dysphagia
Speech problems

Pain control

Pain control can be affected by medical or surgical means. Palliative surgery may assist in pain control, e.g. radical neck dissection, where cure is unlikely. Extensive surgery is rarely indicated. The majority of patients will have satisfactory control of pain by medical treatment or by peripheral nerve block.

Medical control of pain

Medical control of pain is the preferred option, provided the side-effects can be tolerated. Any analgesic preparation prescribed should:

- be appropriate to the degree of pain
- avoid sedation
- have a long duration of action
- be given regularly at an individually determined dose
- preferably be administered orally.

In the early stages, mild analgesics such as aspirin and paracetamol may suffice. However, narcotics should be

Table 2 Use of drugs in the control of pain in terminal head and neck neoplasia	
Nature/source of pain	Analgesic
Lancinating, stabbing	Carbamazepine
Nerve compression	Corticosteroid and narcotic
Muscle spasm	Diazepam
Bone pain	Non-steroid anti-inflammatory drugs (NSAID)
	Radiotherapy

employed as soon as needed. The commonest of these is morphine as an oral preparation. Sublingual and suppository routes for narcotics will be more appropriate in patients with swallowing difficulties.

It is always important to try to determine the underlying aetiology of any pain. This will allow the correct choice of analgesic, as in some cases a simple increase in narcotics will not produce the desired effect and other preparations may be necessary (Table 2).

Radiotherapy appears to be very effective in abolishing pain due to bone involvement.

Surgical control of pain

Non-curative surgery is occasionally considered in alleviating the severe pain of head and neck malignancy. For such cases, reconstructive procedures using myocutaneous flaps may be needed to cover surgical defects. The major cosmetic insult, and the detrimental psychological effect combined with the resectability of the tumour may make such palliative surgery undesirable.

More frequently employed are procedures to denervate the peripheral nervous system. The head and neck is served primarily by the trigeminal, glosopharyngeal, vagus and upper cervical nerves. Destructive procedures may thus provide a satisfactory level of pain relief (Table 3).

Table 3 Source of pain and potential nerve involvement	
Site of pain	Nerve involvement
Skin of face, scalp, mouth, anterior tongue	Trigeminal
Tongue base, tonsil, middle ear	Glossopharyngeal
Oropharynx, hypopharynx, larynx and oesophagus	Vagus
Skin of neck, throat	Upper cervical

Denervation can be produced by percutaneous injection of phenol and alcohol into the nerve near its sensory root. More recently, radiofrequency coagulation has provided an alternative to chemical denervation. On occasion a posterior fossa craniectomy may be employed to allow surgical division of the trigeminal, glossopharyngeal and vagus nerves.

Respiratory difficulties

Respiratory difficulties may arise from physical obstruction of the airway, parenchymal disease in the lung (most patients have smoked heavily) or a feeling of breathlessness from anxiety.

Tumour invasion of the trachea or bronchi producing obstruction may require local radiotherapy, or a bypass tube (tracheostomy, tracheal stent). Costicosteroids can temporarily improve oedema and buy time, and may be used with large doses of opiates if no intervention is planned.

Chest infections are common. Debilitated patients in bed who may have laryngeal overpill and aspiration are particularly at risk. Those with an existing tracheostomy have difficulty in clearing secretions from their chest.

In cases of anxiety, opiates or sedative antidepressant drugs are particularly useful.

Dysphagia

Difficulty in swallowing may be due to local causes such as malignancy or pain from candidal infection. The production of saliva is reduced after radiotherapy and, combined with poor action of the tongue or pharynx, may preclude a solid diet. It is usually possible with the help of a dietitian to discover the type and consistency of food that a patient finds easiest to swallow. Any candidiasis should be treated aggressively, and the addition of benzydamine helps many patients.

Mouth care is essential. This should include regular oral toilet. Sucking ice cubes helps alleviate the feeling of thirst. Dysphagia may be improved by using a short course of corticosteroids.

With progression of the disease, the nutritional status deteriorates. Support in the form of tube or parenteral feeding may be discussed but is usually deemed inappropriate.

Speech problems

Communication difficulties are frequent and naturally will demoralize the patient. The problem is reduced somewhat by continuity of care, so that the patient is not constantly having to adjust to new carers.

It may be beneficial to seek the advice of a speech therapist. They can provide skills to improve communication and in some cases relevant mechanical or electronic aids to speech.

Miscellaneous problems

In the terminal stage of head and neck cancer, the patient may have a number of problems that should be addressed and managed to improve physical and psychological comfort (Table 4).

Table 4 **Distressing problems in terminal head and neck cancer**
Foul smell
Fungating tumour
Mouth and wound infection
Constipation
Pressure necrosis

Necrotic tissue and anaerobic infections combine to produce a foul odour. Treatment of the infection with metronidazole and regular wound toilet usually help reduce the offensive smell. Fungating tumour is unsightly, frequently foul smelling due to infection and may bleed. Regular toilet is essential, but often these patients die from massive sudden haemorrhage, e.g. carotid blow-out (Fig. 1).

Wound and mouth care is mandatory. The regularity of toilet is more important than the methods or materials used (Fig. 2). Sponges soaked with antiseptic are very useful in cleaning dried saliva and food debris, and give a refreshing feel to the mouth.

The combination of regular administration of narcotics, recumbency and general cachexia increases the risks of developing constipation. This can be avoided by the use of aperients, e.g. lactulose.

Pressure skin necrosis occurs in cases of terminal cancer due to a combination of poor nutrition, immobility and loss of control of urinary and bowel sphincters. Good nursing care should prevent problems with pressure areas (Fig. 3).

Role of palliative chemotherapy

Chemotherapy may be considered for patients with advanced disease in whom curative therapy is not an option. The aim of treatment is to improve the quality of life by reducing tumour bulk and hence symptoms, without affecting a cure. The timing of palliative chemotherapy may be difficult. It should not be considered if the patient is asymptomatic or is gaining satisfactory relief of symptoms with other less toxic methods.

There are several contraindications to chemotherapy (Table 5). It is feasible to improve nutritional status and correct other factors so that previously unsuitable patients may be considered for palliative chemotherapy.

Most chemotherapeutic regimens are given in recommended doses at certain intervals of time. Multiagent regimens appear not to confer any greater benefit than the use of single agents.

The major acute side-effects of chemotherapy are nausea and vomiting, but other toxicities are not uncommon and may prevent continuation of therapy (Table 6).

Terminal care — where?

The institution in which the patient is cared for during the terminal illness should be discussed with both the patient and family. Care at home, with a supportive family and nursing care provided by Macmillan or Marie Curie services, may be appropriate. Other possibilities include hospices, e.g. St. Christopher's, who are specially skilled in caring for the dying. Hospital personnel can provide the initial support, prior to the patient going home or to a hospice, but should always be willing to readmit the patient should the situation demand.

Table 5 **Contraindications to palliative chemotherapy**
Severe debilitation
Inadequate renal, liver or cardiac function
Bone marrow suppression

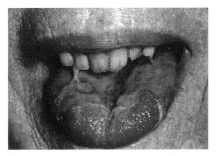

Fig. 2 **A poorly cared for mouth in a patient with terminal head and neck neoplasia.**

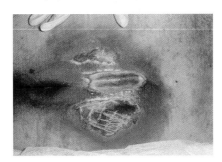

Fig. 3 **Sacral necrosis in a terminally ill patient.**

Table 6 **Toxicity of agents used in palliative chemotherapy**	
Toxicity	**Chemotherapeutic agent**
Renal suppression	Cisplatin
	Methotrexate
Bone marrow suppression	Methotrexate
	5-Fluorouracil
Lung fibrosis	Bleomycin
Mucositis	Methotrexate

> ### Terminal care
>
> - Advanced head and neck malignancy produces major physical and psychological symptoms.
>
> - Pain control is essential in terminal head and neck cancer. This can be provided by medical or surgical means. Breakthrough pain should not be allowed to occur.
>
> - Some degree of relief from dysphagia and respiratory problems can be provided by simple medical means.
>
> - Radiotherapy should be considered to reduce the symptoms due to bone pain or fungating cancer.
>
> - Palliative chemotherapy may prolong survival but has major side-effects and is only rarely indicated.
>
> - Consider carefully where the dying patient will be most appropriately cared for — hospital, hospice or home.

Fig. 1 **A fungating tumour in the neck.** The carotid artery lies in the depth of the mass and may result in a blow out.

Index